# The Food Ain't the Problem

The Food Ain't The Problem
Copyright © 2015 by Carole Holliday
Printed in the United States of America

ISBN 978-0-692-54584-3

Scripture quotations taken from the New American Standard Bible®,
Copyright © 1960, 1962, 1963, 1968, 1971, 1972, 1973, 1975, 1977, 1995 by The Lockman Foundation.
Used by permission. (www.Lockman.org)

Entries taken from the NEW AMERICAN STANDARD EXHAUSTIVE CONCORDANCE®,
© Copyright 1981, 1998 by The Lockman Foundation. Used by permission. (www.Lockman.org)

First Printing, 2015

Carole Holliday c/o Happy Holliday Books
P.O. Box 324
Glendale, CA 91209
TheFoodAintTheProblem@gmail.com

Cover design and illustrations by Carole Holliday
Typesetting/book design by Jennie Lodien (www.jennielodien.com)

*For Robin with her patience and for Carol who cried:*
May we all one day look like our Father.

# Contents

# Acknowledgements
## Deciphering the Chicken Scratch

Writing a book is a lonely endeavor . . . at least it should be. Otherwise there would be no singleness of vision. It's a lot of time and effort, self-doubting and patience. Yet from its solitary birth a book becomes a community experience; one that could be a total disaster if I was presumptuous and just went out there and said "Hey anybody want to read this? Oh . . . wait. Is that a typo?"

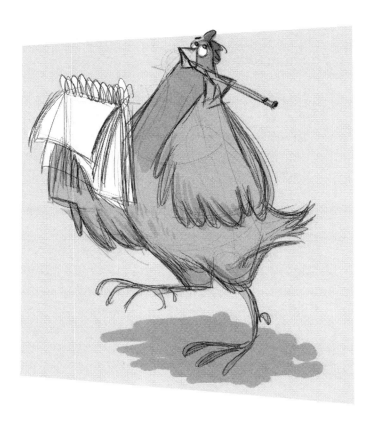

As much as I spent a lot of time writing this massive missive, I'd be a fool if I thought I did this all alone.

The content of this book is drawn from a collection of blog entries, Facebook posts and random thoughts from scraps of paper. It took me nearly as long to write as it did to lose the large chunk of my weight. Ugh.

Thank you, Kathryn Deering, for your cheerful, assiduous editing. Because of your thoroughness people beyond my friends will be able to read my writing.

It turns out there's actually an art to helping the audience be visually comfortable while reading a book. Thank you, Jennie Lodien, for typesetting my finished work. Because of you my book actually looks like one! It's like staggering across the finish line after a grueling a half-marathon and finding an unexpected friend with a prize. Your kindness was God's provision and my heart overflows with gratitude for your generosity.

Speaking of friends: it is touching and interesting to note that the biggest exhorters to write a book to glorify God and His work in my life were two of my non-Christian friends. You encouraged me to go the distance. Thank you. While I will not name you, the Lord knows who you are. My prayer is that someday you'll come to know Jesus Christ as your Savior. You saw enough value in this message to push me to get it out — but it is nothing compared to the God who inspired me to live it. This life is difficult, God knows, but it will be worse if we pass into eternity outside His provision of protection. On this side of death there are worries of the world, but on the other side there is the wrath of God. Please don't face it alone. Your kindness encouraged me, let me encourage you: consider your need and run to Jesus as your Savior. I'm grateful you read my blog, listened to me talk, and encouraged me to finish this task when I grew bored "even if it only helps one or two people." They have you to thank for these assembled words and drawings.

Thank you to Hannah Kaleebi for reading and correcting my fat storage for dummies to make sure I didn't look dumb. I'd like to thank Lisa Hughes who curated my "sermon note" drawings and let me borrow them to supplement the ones I had from my blog, *Cartoons and Cookies*. When I was coerced—ahem, I mean convinced—to add drawings, I almost cried at the thought; it was going to take for-EV-er. Thankfully I remembered she had saved most of the drawings I gave Pastor Jack after his sermons . . . which was an honor and HUGE relief!

Thank you, Julie Martin. You have always been an encouragement. I'm so thankful for your gracious offer to do the last tedious task of proofreading the book and writing my back cover copy. Thank you for sharing what you liked with Ian. It was an honor to know there is something worth passing on. I am grateful to my humble friend Brian Young for cutting down my "Food for Thoughts" to bite-sized chunks. Thanks, also, Jesse Rodriguez for your counsel and guidance regarding my cover design. You pushed me past settling on what I thought was perfect—even changing my title. We are told not to judge a book by its cover— I am glad you reminded me that people will do just that. I'm so happy with the results.

*Lastly,* thank you Jeff Learned and Elizabeth Killian for reading this book. You were my gateway between myself and my readers. You helped me convey my ideas accurately.

As a Christian, it's no big deal to be a bad writer, but it is a horrible thing to put words into the mouth of God. James 3:1 admonishes that not many should become teachers. I don't want to be a teacher. I just want to talk about how awesome God is and how He changed my life. But in so doing, I end up saying, *"Follow my example and do these things I have done . . ."* It makes me a teacher—albeit an unwilling one. I may be lighthearted in my delivery, but I take the message very seriously and don't ever, EVER want to say anything that God didn't say. Proverbs 30:6 says, *"Do not add to His words or He will reprove you, and you will be proved a liar."* In my desire to help anyone who wants to get to the root of their weight problem, I do not want to add anything God has not intended: not just because of fear of reprisal, or embarrassment, but most importantly because I don't want to harm anyone with bad theology. We're desperate to get better, but what does it profit if we get better in our physical lives at the expense of the truth? So my deepest gratitude to you, Beth and Jeff, who sat down with this big fat book with your sword of the truth to correct anything that may have been unintentionally misrepresentative about God.

# Preface:
## My Water Cooler Commissioning

First of all, let me start by saying: *this isn't a diet book*.
There.

Before 2009, I'd been overweight since I was a wee little girl growing up in the 'hood.

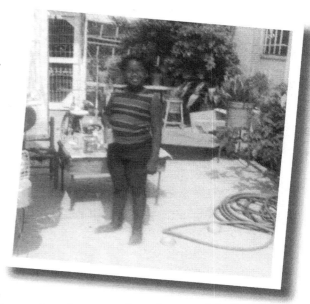

I had a large appetite as a little bitty baby, but it was kept in check until I was six years old and my parents divorced. Let's just say my great Aunt Francis, who took care of my sister and me when my mom was thrust back into the workforce, was a fantastic cook who subscribed to the adage that food is love. By the time I was nine, my mother was shopping in the women's section for my back-to-school wardrobe and it went on from there. The initial pronouncement of baby fat gave way to "your daughter needs to lose weight" and thus began the endless stream of various weight loss attempts. Shock therapy, once-a-week group sessions, and various nasty pre-packaged food programs were all attempted. Not to mention eating only protein or then eating only low fat—or even only juicing. I was ashamed, but not enough to keep it off. As I hit my twenties and into my thirties, there were four times when I got almost to "my goal weight"—each one because of a man I was interested in—but when it didn't pan out, the weight came back and then some. By time I was at my zenith of immensity, I was circus huge and it looked like that was going to be the way I was going to end my days.

I'm sure if you're reading this book the cycle sounds familiar. Even if you don't have a great Aunt Frank or my reasons of loss, loneliness, greed and self-gratification, you have a similar story of habits that put on your pounds. You have an equally similar story of trying to take and keep them off—with no success and great frustration. It's a universal problem. Work up the gumption to lose the weight, have a little success then give up, only to gain more. The Bible says no temptation has overtaken us but such is common to man (1 Cor. 10:13). I just did a quick Amazon search and discovered 27,549 results for weight loss books; everyone wants to lose weight and everyone has ideas on how to do it. Frankly all of them work, yet none of them work at all. People like myself just get fatter and fatter. Sigh.

I work in animation. Very early in my career, I asked a young vice president how he'd achieved his status so early in life. He replied that when he was twenty-six he wanted more opportunities at work but was discouraged by the thought of two more years of school to get an MBA. Unable to make the decision, he did what any smart young man should do—he asked an older wise man for counsel:

"You're concerned that if you take two years to get your MBA you'll be twenty eight years old when you're done? How old will you be in two years if you don't get your MBA?"

Over the years, I've often thought about that story when it came to addressing being fat. I'd think, "I really should do something about this issue no matter how long it takes to lose, because in the end the time is going to pass whether or not I deal with it . . ." So I'd work really hard and lose the weight for a while, but then:

Bwooink!
   Why hello there, Back Fat.
      Where have you been Hip Saddlebags?

Grrrumble . . . oh well. Might as well go ahead and eat that second pizza.

I'd gain it back and then some . . . okay—a lot.

So why try? It seems pretty hopeless and, frankly, like a lot of hard work over a long time to tenuously, bitterly hang on to victory—*if* there's victory. And if there's no victory (which is more often the case) to be rewarded with not only more fat, but also a large helping of shame and self-remorse on the side.

Yet God showed me a way to walk through the forest of my struggles and helped me lose 150 pounds. He also showed me how to recover when I fell off the wagon, instead of giving up.

So here I am, writing a book on a topic that causes frustration and shame. I'm writing a book about something that's been covered so many times by people more medically adroit, physically capable or perhaps more spiritually educated than me . . . Why?

First of all I realized that losing weight is not the issue in losing weight. I saw God was more concerned about something far more ugly than my muffin top, stretch marks, back boobs and love handles. In fact, He was so concerned about it, He slaughtered His only Son to show me just how much He hated this thing that caused me so much emotional, physical, sociological and most importantly, spiritual destruction—all the while being crazy-over-the-top in love with me, whom He had created for a purpose and a hope.

Does this thought get your attention? I hope so, because at the beginning of my exodus from the land of fat, it got mine. As I fought through this journey through the jungle like an intrepid explorer with a machete, I learned quite a few things that I wrote on blog posts, social media status updates and scraps of paper. I had conversations that people would remind me of later and I dictated thoughts into my phone. But write a book? Ugh, it was enough work losing the weight, please, please, please, don't make me work more by having to track back through the breadcrumbs of ideas and turn them into a book. For the love of everything holy: let my blog be enough! Pretty please with a cherry on top?

I see now that, like Jonah, I was called for a purpose even though, like Jonah, I wanted to run from it. Yet who can resist the will of God? Especially when He speaks to you from an unlikely source.

The tipping point came when I'd been asked to give my testimony at a women's retreat of how God motivated me to gradually lose the weight. The following Monday while standing near the coffee machine, I told one of my good friends at work that people said I should write a book after I'd read my testimony to the room full of women. My friend rolled his eyes in a "Yeah, duh, obviously" attitude, assuming I meant something

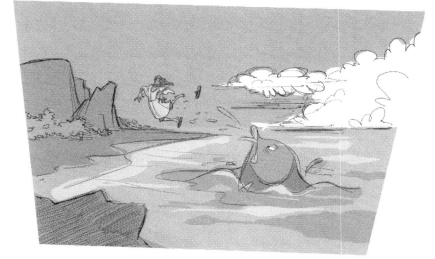

fictional, or maybe finally the romantic comedy script I was procrastinating about doing.

"No not that kind of writing—they meant something else."

My friend, always the encourager, went on with an "okay, I'll bite" tone in his voice. "So . . . why do they think you should write?"

"They want me to write on weight loss, and frankly I think it's silly. I mean there are so many books out there on how to lose weight and all of them would work if people would just do them, what's the point of writing one more?'

My friend flipped the lever of the coffee dispenser and was genuinely interested.

"What did you say?"

In the nanoseconds between hearing the question and actually responding to it, a number of thoughts flashed through my mind. You see, this friend is agnostic. It was a challenge to be vulnerable with a room full of loving, smiling women who looked at me with kindness and acceptance, but with him, my response became more complicated. Do I tell him my testimony? Do I share the gospel? Will he think it's silly? Will he say it's a crutch? The brain is a wonderfully lightning-fast computer; as I went through those questions, I simultaneously thought of the one time a few months before when I had actually shared the gospel with him and he laughed at me and walked away. The image of him turning on his heels and heading back to his office was burned into my mind and it made me apprehensive—and yet, this was a chance to talk about the God I loved so much to a friend about whom I cared so much.

I hastily told him what I had told the women, how God had changed my heart through believing in the gospel and had given me the power to not diet, but still lose weight anyway by obeying what He showed me in the Bible. Then I braced myself for his even-hastier exit.

My friend didn't retreat. Instead he got a strange look on his face like someone had poked him, and then he blurted out:

"You need to write that . . . I never thought of it that way before . . . Even if it helps one or two people, you need to write that down . . ."

*Wait, what?* I thought, *But you're not saved. By your own admission you have no time for God* . . . Yet here was this man telling me I needed to write a book that would bring the very God (whose rule he shunned) into the spotlight to show Him for all His beauty and love for His creation He had sacrificed all to buy back from slavery and death.

It was a game changer. *It's a bit daunting, because though I have lost most of my weight, I have yet more to go* . . . As I start this book, I'm re-losing the last of the 36 pounds I gained over the summer (well, at least it wasn't 150). Shouldn't I be done, with my fists in the air like Rocky, before I can point to the faithfulness of God? But the Spirit reminded me of the apostle Paul's words to the church in Philippi:

> *Not that I have already obtained it or have already become perfect, but I press on so that I may lay hold of that for which also I was laid hold of by Christ Jesus. Phil. 3:12*

So here I am writing a book on submission to God because in the end, a nonbeliever told me I had to.

Weight is my struggle, and, if you've picked up this book, it's yours as well. Someone who's perfect didn't write this book; it's written by someone who's loved by a gracious God and who's being led to walk in obedience. If you do the things in this book you will find success over time. But more importantly, I hope you'll find the greater treasure of how much God loves you.

Through the course of this book I'll unpack the thoughts I had while losing my weight. Various friends have tried to encourage me that reading a book like this will give others hope as I share my struggles so they can identify with me. While that may be true, I realize it can backfire. You see, while our struggles may be the same, I realize we're all unique.

Years ago when I was working on a film project for a studio, I went to a local agricultural college for a day trip to research a day in the life of an Old Testament Hebrew shepherd. While I was there, I went out with the shepherd on duty as he walked the sheep from their holding area to where they were to go for that part of the day. There was something kind of fun and sweet about standing above a crowd of medium-sized puffballs with little spindly legs that looked largely the same as they bustled in a tight pack on their way, heads down. Strangely, the one thing that struck me was as we meandered across the dusty ground: the blanket of noise and sheep-sounds gave way to individual voices—some high, some strangely low, some thin and whiny, others rich and full—all coming from these fluffballs that really had nothing else to distinguish them one from the other. I remarked to the shepherd that their uniqueness of voices astonished me. They all looked the same, and yet they all sounded so different. The shepherd replied, "Yes, the shepherd knows the voice of his sheep."

Jesus is called the Good Shepherd. John 10:3 says that He calls the sheep by name and leads them. Imagine that—the God of the universe who spoke into existence these worlds that function with the intricate precision of the finest clock is a Shepherd who not only made all this, but can see all the individual parts as they function and knows them uniquely.

He knows you.

He knows me.

So if He knows our unique voices as we cry out in the crowd of people who look largely the same, why would we think that the solution to our problems would be any less unique to our own individual selves? I'll talk a little of my struggles if it's an encouragement for you to know you're not the only one who ever ate an entire cake in one sitting, but in the end, that's not what changed me, seeing other people struggle with the same things I did. What changed me was learning that God saw me and loved me.

God saw me . . .

He didn't want to change who I was personally. He made me with a purpose and like any artist, He delighted in all the things that made me, me. However what He did want to change was my sin. There were attitudes, actions and habits that marred His creation of me. Those things, He wanted to remove so that I would actually be the very best version of my-self: the Carole Holliday who reflects the image of Christ. What you will be reading therefore is not a one-size-fits-all approach to Christian weight loss. As children of an infinitely creative God, our voices are entirely different. That's why I believe in the Bible; God doesn't focus on our externals so much as our hearts that make our unique voices unique. Even

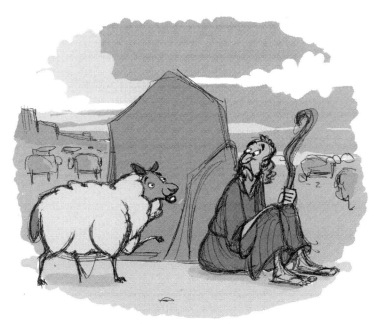

I dig the bucolic scene like the next guy, but lets rap about the meaning of life, man.

though this book hits on the aspects of what I did to lose the weight—my approach to food, exercise, and where I found my heart to change—I hope it will lead you to something greater: a re-alization of how much God loves His creation of you because there is no other like you.

While I am insisting on the idea we need to delight that Jesus knows our voice, that's not enough. I hope that the words of this sheep named Carole will be a megaphone to amplify the voice of the Shepherd who laid down His life for you and for me. In the end, with all our uniqueness, we'll be before the throne of God marveling at Him for all eternity. No words of mine can even come close to the reality of the one we will finally see to worship with clarity, like someone in love trying to explain why the object of their affection has captured their interest and yet they try, not because they think their description will do the lover justice, but because that person exists. God exists, and that reality should change our lives. He will be the focus of our eternity.

Above all, this book will have a decidedly Christian slant. I wish I could say God has the corner on self-improvement, but that's not the case. Yes, non-Christian people lose weight every day. Sometimes they're even horrible people with awful, vindictive personalities. One has only to turn on the television or flip open a magazine to see the biggest, fattest, extremist makeover before-and-after transformations, to see that a life with Christ isn't the only life that promises a better outcome in this area. I've had non-Christian people tell me it was all because of my hard work, willpower and determination that I got to where I am. No protes-tation of mine that it was God's work and direction that guided that determination could make them change their minds.

Yes, people can drastically change their external appearance if they put their minds to it. *However, only God can change a person's heart.*

The understanding that God's loving heart surgery is the source of your weight trans-formation is what I'll seek to offer in the pages of this book. Because when the last bit of confetti has been swept from the stage, and people have gotten used to your new and improved size and no longer compliment you on all your hard work—there will still be that gnawing feeling of fear and emptiness about all you've accomplished. In the end, the relative short-term goal of a healthier life that inspired all the hard work, determination and self-denial proves to be empty. Because when the chips finally fall as they may, what you realize is that it doesn't matter if you're healthier, if you find that for as long as you walk this earth you're saddled with bearing this enormous burden of change all alone.

# A Note About the Art . . .

When I told my friends I was begrudgingly writing a book on weight loss, in their enthusiastic excitement they would invariably ask, "of course you're going to illustrate it, right?"

Excuse me, why?

Because you're an artist.

But what does that have to do with losing weight?

While they couldn't come up with a satisfactory answer to my question as to why they wanted to make more work for me, I finally decided to cave into their whims and add doodles and drawings I created for various sources during my five-year weight transformation journey to this book because . . . well, after all, I am an artist.

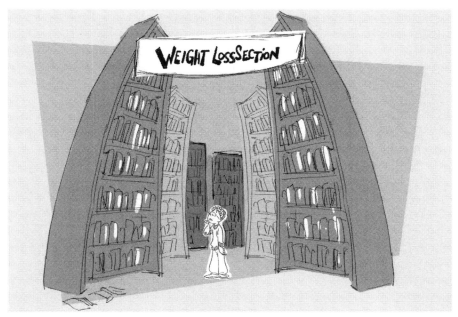

"So there is nothing new under the sun.
Is there anything of which one might
say, 'See this, it is new?'
Already it has existed for ages
which were before us."
ECC. 1:9.10

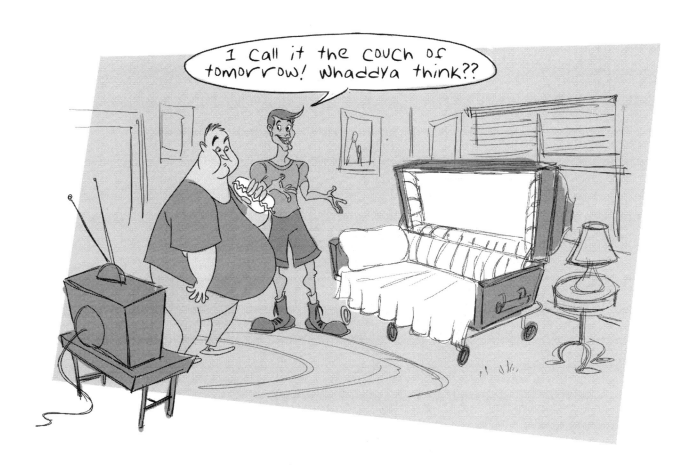

# Prologue:
## To the Thins Wherever You Are

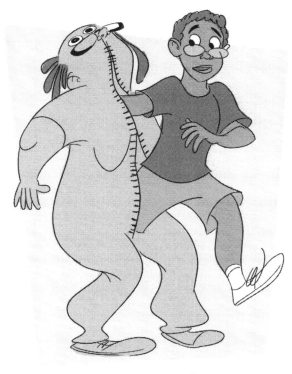

As easy as?

I know it seems random, but when I started this journey down from 312 pounds to where I am today, I told myself at the end of each successful day in obeying God in all the things He was teaching me concerning my appetite, that before His throne in heaven I was a size six. Okay—admittedly that might have been a bit much, but I took the idea from the Bible where the apostle Paul refers to the Christians he wrote to as "saints," although they were far from perfected and needed to learn so much. I decided that I too should no longer identify myself by what I once was, even if from time to time I stumbled. This is a book for those who are Thins: children of God whom He's empowered to overcome their sin which leads to long-term weight gain. Paul didn't stop at telling those who believed the message of Christ that they were saints, he told them what was expected of them in their new identity. Like Paul, I want to encourage you who read this book about what will be expected of you in being a "Thin."

One morning while at the gym I told a personal trainer about my plans to write a book on weight loss. He listened guardedly when I told him how the book would focus more on repentance and internal heart change rather than only the conventional drive to emphasize workouts and nutrition. Finally he said, "Well, remember culturally some people would think its rude not to eat a lot." As he spoke on worldwide cultural acceptances for our various eating habits I told him about Don Richardson, a missionary, who moved his family to minister to a tribe of people who thought violence, deceit and murder were culturally acceptable. In fact, when that tribe first heard the story of Jesus, they thought *Judas* was the hero and lauded his ability for being able to vanquish Jesus by his cunning deceit. Their opinion was changed when Don Richardson explained that Jesus was no ordinary man and in fact was sent by God to create peace with mankind similar to the way that tribe used a "peace child" to avert war between their tribe and others around them. In light of understanding the identity of Christ, the tribe could see Judas' deceitful betrayal of his friend and teacher for the evil that it was.

The trainer acquiesced to the example of how living by culture can prove destructive but went on to say his goal in helping people lose their weight was to get them not to think about looking better, but to feel better about being able to do more. I applauded him for his desire to change his clients' minds, but added that my goal went deeper. My goal was to pave a way to change a person's heart, and a heart can only be changed by finding hope that despite how broken, inconsistent and petty it is, the person who owns it will still be loved. I told him in no uncertain terms that God was the answer to that change of heart, because God's love forgives and points a way out of the darkness that's not based on feelings but based on His unflinching and impeccable character.

God's love working through God's character supernaturally empowers us emotionally, as well as physically, to persevere through anything He calls us to do. And that hope of being protected, guided, strengthened and comforted produces more than just will power and determination—it produces gradual and lasting genuine transformation, inside and out. In the case of the contents of this book, a person motivated in this way finds that by following God he or she not only melts the fat in their cells, they are able to endure in the times when they do it less than perfectly, resting in the knowledge that the ugliest part of them won't be judged, but instead lovingly transformed for the better.

Even though in the end my trainer and I disagreed on what provided lasting results, his words still made me think—there can be cultural differences in how we eat. In today's Western culture some people would say eating too much is okay if love is involved, or if they think you look too thin. Other people say we need to watch our weight so we can live healthier, longer lives. Still others would say we need to eat certain ways because science "tells us to"—until science "tells us to" something else a few years later. In the end, it changes with the passage of time and man's often uninformed or emotion-based, evolving opinions. People are fickle creatures who go by looks, feelings and their limited understanding. However, God is above culture. He's trustworthy because He's perfect, knows everything, is unaffected by emotional whims and never changes who He is. Wouldn't it make sense to base your catalyst for change on someone who knows the beginning from the end and dependably stays the same no matter what you throw at Him, instead of a manmade system that varies with the whims of people who change their minds depending on their latest discoveries? I want to encourage anyone who reads this (all two of you) that God knows how we are best to function. If we agree with His standards as outlined in the Bible, we'll reset to how He intends us to best perform.

The implications are far-reaching: In this postmodern age in which one culture asserts one idea while a different culture espouses another, I'm relieved that Jesus is the same yesterday, today and tomorrow and His Word never changes. This applies to everything from weight loss to navigating relationships. It applies to all the struggles that are common to mankind in all its dimensions. Following God's commands we see that what we once thought were seemingly matter-of-fact statements are actually declarations of God's love to the people He's created.

In tackling the reasons for our weight gain, we need to focus beyond what culture says to what God shows us. Some of it will make perfect sense, while some of it might leave us scratching our heads. God's ways aren't our ways, nor His thoughts our thoughts, but that's what makes His commandments so very hopeful. I know that If I had to rely on my own limited intelligence to solve my myriad of problems, I'd only get so far, the hole I'm in is too deep and my strength is inadequate. But in God, who is infinite in all His attributes, there's a permanent way of escape from all the hopelessness that exists in our own unique situations. It is a way we'd never see on our own, not if we sat and looked for it for a million years.

I hope this book encourages you that even if you never make it before you die to the "Metropolitan Life Height/Weight Scale" ideal for how much you should weigh, God is concerned that you live your life in the light of what He's revealed for you and He's pleased, not because you look or feel better, but because you're striving to obey Him. Confessing your failings and falling in line with His ways doesn't always feel pleasurable at first, but in the long run, it ends up feeling REALLY great and the life you gain for obeying God goes far beyond your wildest imagining.

Are you willing to take that leap of faith into the unknown with the encouragement that though the way is a mystery to you, there is a loving God waiting to catch you?

This journey I'm outlining in the pages of this book isn't a quick-fix process. I've come to see as I've stumbled along, five steps forward and one and a half steps

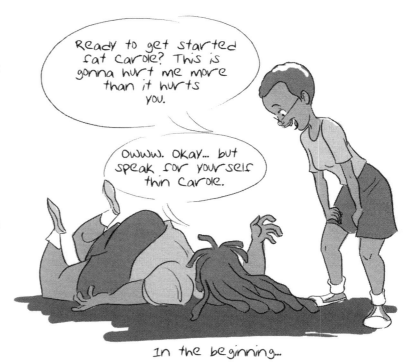

In the beginning...

back, that the progression of turning this aspect of my life over to His control is as much about patience as it is about self-control and physical discipline. The world wants to lose weight fast and often does. On the other hand, though following God's commands may prove to beget slower external results, I beg you to understand that your outward results might be slow because God is busy building some aspect of your inward character, like installing supports for a high-rise. God intends the building He does in us to weather all storms and last into the eternity He gives us after we die, so His work inside our hearts is more important to Him than getting us in record time to the number on the scale we have in mind.

Therefore the first part of this book will focus on structural issues. It's only the last four chapters that will tell you what I did to lose the weight. DON'T. SKIP. AHEAD! I only tell you about the book structure because you might start thinking as you fan through the pages of this book, "I thought this was a weight loss book . . .what's with all this God stuff?" Rest assured, all this "God stuff" is how I was able to tackle the problem of weight and execute the last six chapters of the book. Without knowing how to understand Him, His love, and what He considers the problem for why I packed on the pounds, I was doomed to remain porcine.

At the writing of this book I was training to hike Mount Whitney that at 14,505 feet is the tallest mountain in the contiguous United States. Fearful I wasn't going to be able to handle the altitude and long, steady climb, I hired a more specialized trainer who was formerly a mountain guide. His exercises were non-conventional; designed not to make me look beautiful, but to give me power and control even though at times I found myself thinking "Uh, yeah, right—what's the purpose of carrying this here and then back again? This is just silly." In addition to the workouts at the gym, I ran long distances and submitted myself weekly to long, punishing hikes, to work on the mental stamina needed to face the twenty-two mile round trip to Whitney's rocky summit and back.

At one point, one of my friends took me to Joshua Tree National Park to help me face my fear of heights by rock climbing. During the weekend, some of us went into a cave. Now if they had told me the cave was actually more like a *cave-in,* then I might have balked at the chance. So here I was, armed with only a headlamp, following the small crowd of mostly high school kids headfirst into this black scramble of tumbled-in boulders and awkward pinch points. Had I not trained with the trainer, though I was now small enough to fit through the narrow spaces, I still would have struggled, because I wouldn't have had the physical strength gained in those random-seeming exercises to pull myself through all the tiny awkward bends and crawls. Furthermore, had I not done the drudgery of long distances I wouldn't have had the mental ability to calm my heart in the relentless darkness. Also when I *did* fall through a space between some of the boulders barely covering a cave underneath, I wouldn't have had the ability to laugh it off, though I would later have a giant bruise on my knee and a thrashed elbow. I was prepared for the unknown challenges I faced in the cave by the slow steady work I had done on my own and with the trainer.

Oftentimes we're prepared for the caves in our lives by the seeming drudgery of God's discipline when we're in the light. This book focuses on how to come to God and be trained. Just like my trainer, who did things that made no sense to me yet I found in the end they yielded unexpected results, God also trains us in ways we may not understand.

The things He calls us to do and change are not to make us miserable. They have a greater purpose. Though they may make our lives better here in the long run, in the end, the things that He asks us to do here are what prepare us for the altitude of heaven, where He Himself is our pinnacle. I hope this book can be a small guide along the way. God's ways are not our ways which is fine with me because His ways prepare us for His kingdom, which bears no resemblance to this broken-down world in which we live!

**So there you have it. Everything that this book will cover: God loves you and has a wonderful plan for your weight. But it's not because he wants you to be a supermodel. He wants you to be ready to come into His eternal kingdom.**

· · · · · · ·

As in any physical change, results may vary. Be patient and committed. Above all, remember that what you are about to read is more than a body makeover—it is a life change.

Oh, and just as a little request: You need to go to your doctor . . . you know, the one you've been avoiding because you don't want to hear the lecture on how you need to lose weight? Please get a physical to make sure you're good to go. While I won't be discussing anything radical (I'm a *cartoonist,* for crying out loud, and no professional in the realm of health, nutrition and exercise), go to your doctor and make sure there's no underlying reason for your weight problem beyond the

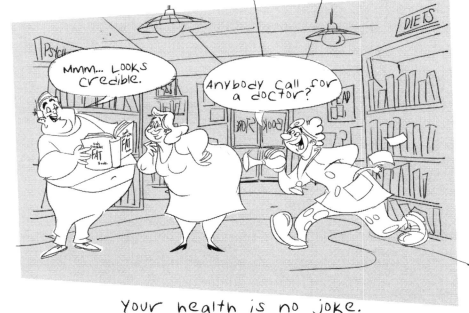

Your health is no joke.

fact that you eat too much. Make sure your doctor is okay with you eating less and moving more. Once you've done that, then you're good to move on from there—if you're healthy, with no excuses, or if you have some limitations, with reasons to proceed with caution. Follow the advice in this book at your own risk. *You're* responsible for your health, *not me.*

As long as we're talking about going to the physician, let me encourage you to go the Great Physician, God Himself. Please take the time to read the included Bible references. It's only by the power of God working through the word of God I was able to affect this change I'm about to unpack for you. If you're tempted to only go with what I've written and skip reading the verses, (in the context of how they're originally intended) you'll miss out on the most important thing. Not weight loss, but having the God of the universe unfold His love for you through His word as it applies to your struggle. Remember, not one sparrow falls without His noticing—He sees you in your frustration and desire to overcome this dauntingly oppressive task.

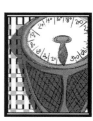

# Take A-Weigh

- God's message transcends man's cultures.
- Lasting change is internal and can take some time.
- Go to a doctor!

# Food for Thought

*❝Every man's way is right in his own eyes, but the Lord weighs the hearts. ❞ Proverbs. 21:2*

In the long run, God is more interested in your HMI than your BMI (body mass index). By HMI, I mean your heart mass index. When our hearts get bloated with the sins we refuse to relinquish, it spills over into our relationships. Everything is affected, from how we interact with God to our jobs, to the government, to each other and even to ourselves. God wants to help us address that which makes our hearts spiritually unhealthy not just so we can shrink our bottoms, but so He can equip us to fly on wings like eagles (Isa. 40:28-31).

Take a little bit of time to weigh your heart before the Lord. Answer these questions honestly. My hope is that as you expose the motivations of your heart and assess your available assets, you'll be more ready to receive what you're about to read over the next 15 chapters.

- **How long have you been overweight and why do you want to lose weight?**

- **Are you willing to commit to changing?**

- **By what methods have you attempted to lose weight in the past?**

- **What's the longest time you've kept off your weight?**

- **Do you live alone, with family/roommates, or with a spouse?**

- **What is your family like? Are they supportive? Are they overweight as well?**

- **Do you have people who support you?**

- **What are some of your favorite "can't live without" foods?**

- **What's your relationship to portion sizes?**

- **What's your relationship to intentional exercise?**

- **Are you an emotional eater?**

- **What's your relationship like with God?**

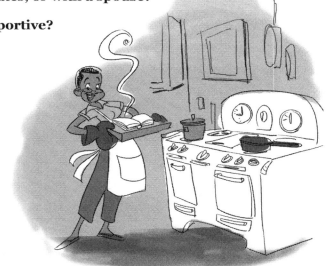

BECAUSE no one ever gained a pound from thinking too much.

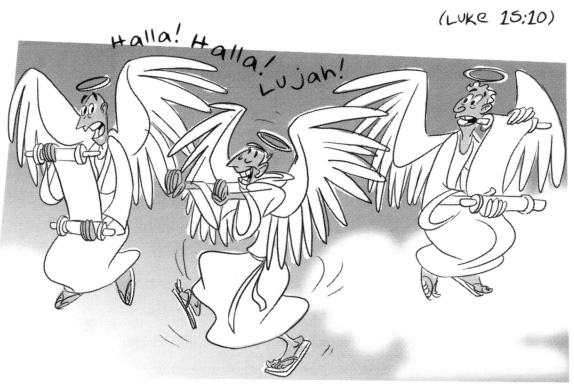

(Luke 15:10)

Angus the avid angel applied sincerity as he celebrated each single sinner's salvation.

Chapter 1

# Charging The Battery

> *For this reason also, since the day we heard of it, we have not ceased to pray for you and to ask that you may be filled with the knowledge of His will in all spiritual wisdom and understanding, so that you will walk in a manner worthy of the Lord, to please Him in all respects, bearing fruit in every good work and increasing in the knowledge of God; strengthened with all power, according to His glorious might, for the attaining of all steadfastness and patience; joyously giving thanks to the Father, who has qualified us to share in the inheritance of the saints in Light.* Colossians 1:9–14

I recently went with some friends on a hiking trip to Zion, Utah. Because I'm afraid of driving on heights, I agreed to carpool on the condition that I share the price of gas. We were excited as we hit the road, so many adventures lay ahead of us from hiking through the ravine of the Narrows along and through the Virgin River, to challenging ourselves to cross the ridiculously skinny land bridge with thousand foot drop-offs on either side to get to Angels Landing. We chattered along happily heading out on our seven-and-a-half-hour drive.

All that happy banter stopped cold when the air conditioner shut off in the desert and several minutes later the car conked out completely just one hour into our journey. The battery in my friend's electric car had died and there was no resurrecting it.

Before we start this "journey of discipline" to our destination of less weight, I want to make sure you've got power to get there.

Great, what's the power?

The message contained in the gospel of Jesus Christ will give you the power to change the way you live. Perpetually taking it to heart will enable you to go the distance in battling any character flaw and as the apostle Paul said in 1 Timothy 4:7, *discipline yourself for the purpose of godliness.*

The contents of this chapter are the reason I was able to live everything you'll read in the rest of *The Food Ain't the Problem*. It's what got me going in the first place and is what continues to be the power, the forgiveness and hope that help get me back on track when I inevitably wander from what God has shown me in the Bible as the right way to successfully battle my weighty issues.

While being fat isn't a sin—yes I said fat; let's call that spade a spade—often the reasons we get fat, if not health-related, have been caused by sin— but more on that later. God gives His children the power to overcome this sin as well as every sin that besets us. To access that power, we need to make sure we are His children.

## To the Two People Reading This Book

You nonbelievers may be tempted to skip this chapter because you don't want to be preached at. You think your life's pretty fine and you're a good person who just happens to be a few pounds overweight, and you hope this book might be the magic bullet to get you over your dietary malaise. You may or may not believe there's a God, and even if there is one, you believe you're good enough and God isn't such a hard-nose that He's going to do anything to you of any extreme and lasting consequence like send you to hell because He looks at your heart and sees that you "mean well." After all, isn't meaning well good enough?

If you're a Christian: the temptation may be to skip this chapter because you know the whole drill. You have all the right words and you can share the message of God's hope with your non-Christian friends like the best of the Christian apologists. But if you're like me, in your heart of hearts you sense that something's missing. You love God, you love the Bible, and yet when faced with choosing between heavenly thoughts and a fourth helping of a loaded pizza, God usually takes a back seat . . . until you try again tomorrow. . .

Okay— well how about next week, because after all, it's Friday and the week's already been a mess anyway.

Sigh . . .

To the one who hasn't heard this message before—or has heard it and rejected it, I hope the simplicity of the good news you're about to read will inspire you to a greater goal than a smaller size. I hope it will change your status from enemy of God to His child. Meanwhile to the believer who knows all this, even if I say nothing you haven't heard already, I pray this is a reminder of how precious you are to God as His child.

God created this world and will one day stand in judgment over it, yet He has a love for mankind that flies high above our human comprehension. Let my attempt to pluck the ineffable from the air and set it on the pages of this chapter be my humble road map to the heart that God has for all of humanity. I pray both nonbeliever and believer alike see His love in this first message, for the gospel is a love story for a brood of rebels. Without understanding it, any attempt at the change offered in the later pages of this book will move forward for a while, but eventually pffffizzle like the columbine flower I put in my back yard which I forgot to water.

# The Good News According to Carole

To begin with: God is.

He's the reason why the birds sing their songs, because He created them, not by explosive chance but by the power of His word. He's the source of all the laws, from the ones that cause an apple to fall to the ground to the ones that show us right from wrong. He's the source of the greatness of humanity: the reason the muscles of the most amazing athlete can power him or her to excel at their given sport, or the reason some scientist can have a flash of brilliance which discovers a cure to make lives better. He's the reason the mountains tower high and the ocean depths are unfathomable. God is the reason you just drew the breath you took, and the next one you will take.

God exists and has His own actions and attitudes. He's far above us as a Being, with abilities far above our own. Just because we can't understand a Being so much different than ourselves, doesn't mean He can't exist. It just means our minds aren't completely equipped to grasp someone outside the scope of all we know. Some people try to explain Him away, which is pretty handy so they don't have to feel badly about their failings, but foolish when it comes to finding help when they're lost.

The acceptance of God's existence is the beginning of all hope (Prov. 1:7, 9:10) because if God is, then God can do all the things He says He can.

In the Bible, the Greek word *euaggelion* is translated into English as the word "gospel" which means good news. It's so easy to take that definition for granted. Like "Hey I just found out I saved money by switching my car insurance" good news, or "I just changed my Facebook status from 'single' to in a 'relationship'" good news. In the cases of our good news, it's temporary. In a world where things fall apart or lose their excitement, the goodness of our good news fades. The cars we insured for less get old, and the relationship we touted as amazing hits the invariable snags and becomes work.

However the Good News of the gospel really truly is good news, because it's based on someone that doesn't rust, fall apart or degenerate. It's based on God who never goes back on His word, never EVER changes and always exists in perfection, *in perpetuity!* Therefore the gospel of God that promises hope and life will always bring light into darkness, and hope into despair. It can be trusted completely because it will always do what it promises; God guarantees it.

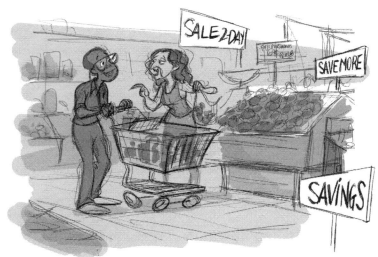

Speaking of savings have you heard that God gave up His only Son so you could be saved from your sins?

The gospel is simple. So simple a child can understand it, yet it's so profound that every time I understand another aspect of it in how it affects my life, my mind's blown all over again. But what exactly is the good news? What is the gospel?

I'm glad you asked . . . *well, I'm glad I asked for you.*

Once upon a time God created man to have a relationship with Him and God was right there with man: walking with him where he could see Him. However man decided that having God walking with him wasn't good enough. Instead, man wanted to be LIKE God so he could run his own life and no threat of death could convince him otherwise. (Gen. 2:15, 3:1-22).

So man took a trade-down: He got access to the wisdom of God (which is like trying to pour the ocean into a thimble) AND for a lovely parting gift, he was now separated from the God who created and loved him. Good times. Parted from God, he was now spiritually dead and would one day be physically dead for all of eternity.

So a bunch of years went by, and the world showed the effects of what it meant to live under man's occupancy. All the bad stuff that's happened on this planet—the stuff we blame on God? That'd be man. All the murders, the lies, the deceptions and thievery. All the wantonness, carousing, hatred and envy, all the broken hearts, broken lives, broken bodies— that's just man living on this earth as his own god. Living life with the knowledge of good and evil, but lacking the ability to properly execute it with consistency because human understanding of what good and evil is changes from culture to culture, epoch to epoch—or even due to what someone had for dinner the night before. Man became as dangerous as a toddler with a gun.

All the while mankind raised their collective fist and said, "If God is so loving, then why'd He allow all this evil to happen?" To which God quietly replies, "because it was your choice."

Man is right; such a god is cruel, murderous and all things evil. However, they refuse to recognize that the god to whom they are referring is the one who looks back at them from their mirrors. Mankind is the god of this life, and human beings are, at their best, the worst of all monsters, and at their worst, the most beautiful of all demons. For centuries, they've died and gone to where demons belong—in an eternal separation from the true God and His beauty, they've gone to hell.

Which, for a God who made man to be loved, is pretty much a heartbreaking concept. What to do? . . . What to do? . . .

How do you win back someone who hates you—especially when they're, you know, spiritually dead? How do you deal with the fact that that very same person must pay an infinitely unpayable price for their mutiny? How to do all this and still remain true to who you are as God who is perfect, holy and has the final word on everything? It's not going to work to say, *"Oh, okay, you win. I love you all too much to let this little bitty thing like your treason to stand between us."* That'd mean God had sunk below man's level in order to accept him— a level that shifts to the lowest common denominator minute by minute. For man with his thimbleful of knowledge, restoring the broken relationship between God and man would be a problem he's powerless to solve, but for God who's the source of all wisdom, He already had a plan.

In lots of countries, a person who renounces their citizenship and sides with the enemy gets the death penalty for their treason. All of humanity is guilty of this treason against God and His eternal heavenly kingdom for rejecting His rule. Veering off the course of God's commands even in one point shows a person's rebellious heart. Everybody misses the mark when it comes to living by God's standards. Even the people who vehemently insist, "I'm a good person—after all I haven't murdered anyone!" Everybody means everybody. Even *you*. Therefore God promises that every rebel will die.

God keeps all His promises, even if the promise is at His own personal expense. He promised death to His created beings and all of their descendants for rejecting His rule, so someone had to die for that rejection. The good news is: That someone doesn't have to be *you*. Jesus, the sinless, perfect God/Man was slaughtered sacrificially in man's place to pay the price of death, which man the traitor had incurred (Rom. 5:6–11). The choice in reading this message is this: Embrace the good news or accept the consequences for rejecting it.

Hell: a place of darkness, torment, loneliness, sorrow and eternal bitterness. No comfort, no reprieve. All this in a perfect and incorruptible body, for all eternity.

Seems pretty extreme, I know. But think about it, really think about it: If we puny humans get bent out of shape when someone cuts us off on the road, wouldn't it stand to reason that thumbing our nose to God Himself by saying "I want *your* place God. I don't want You to rule over me!" would elicit a hellish punishment to suit such a heavenly crime?

# This Hurts He More Than It Hurts You

Hearing you're a sinner bound for eternal torment and separation from God (even if you're a relatively nice person) is alarming. It's a blow to your pride to come to the understanding that God, who is love, doesn't love you as you are and has written your name on hell's fiery ledger. However, hearing this message actually proves just how much God DOES love you, even if His message hurts your feelings to hear.

I was night-hiking on a narrow trail when I lost my footing and fell. A man behind me grabbed my arm as I went down, and I landed gracelessly on my bottom. In the limited revelation of the light that I had from my headlamp, I decided I would just scoot down to the next level, unaware that when I'd fallen, I'd gotten disoriented and was now going to scoot off a cliff! In the dark I couldn't tell I was in danger and in fact tried a couple times to go that direction even though my rescuer kept telling me no. It dawned on me that maybe there was a reason he was blocking my choice and I realized I wasn't even on the path. I thanked him for saving me by any means possible. Sure my shoulder was injured (and would hurt for several months after) but I am thankful to be alive. That's the love of God in the gospel: pulling each and every one of us from walking off the cliff and setting our feet on the right path, even though we think we know the way.

How does God pull a person from the cliff? You know how everyone says that God is love? This is the part that makes people who fight against God's penalty of hell get their undies in a bunch. "If God can be love," they say, "then how can He send me to hell if I'm working on being a good person?" But you need to understand that your self-proclaimed "good" is not good enough. God who's perfect demands nothing short of *perfection*. In this, you're either walking on the path or you're walking off it. So this is where God is love: Not in giving us what we want, but in giving us what we need. We may find we hurt, but it saves our lives. For God to stoop to accept "good enough" as "enough" wouldn't be possible, since it's so unlike Him. Like the time I was helping a teacher friend correct some spelling tests and the little girl got all of the words right except for the word "receive." She had done so well, I asked my friend, "can't we just give it to her anyway?" I have no idea why I asked that; the word was still wrong, even if every other word was spelled correctly.

So God, because He is love, made peace with this treasonous world by a way that would both save mankind and allow God to keep His perfect standard. Jesus, being born of a human and born of God, came to solve the problem. As a man, He could be tempted by all the things that caused man to commit treason, but as God, He could withstand falling to that temptation. So when an angry mob, still thinking they knew what was right for themselves and this world, nailed Him to a cross, Jesus with His lifetime of perfection at that moment became the hand to reach out to pull all mankind from their plunge over the cliff into a godless, painful oblivion.

Jesus died after living a perfect and sinless life. He died publicly in front of family, followers and foes alike. Jesus was God, yet still a man bound by the laws of the earth: Gravity pulled at Him while He miraculously healed the sick, ultraviolet rays from the sun baked his skin and turned him brown in the summers as He explained the Scriptures as no human teacher could. Lack of food caused his stomach to grumble while He shared the good news with the unlovely, and dehydration on the cross caused him to thirst while He uttered the words "Father, forgive them, for they know not what they are doing." And death? Well it stopped all of those things instantly. He died. Like all men ever have, or ever will.

Jesus the God/Man died.

He died, but He didn't stay dead.

Because God the Father did the most fantastical thing!

God the Father, with His ocean-full of wisdom and the power to do something about it, demonstrated His ultimate power. He built a bridge between Himself and this world that had decided they didn't need Him when He raised Jesus from the dead. God filled Jesus' lungs with air; He caused his heart to pump blood though His circulatory system; He caused His muscles to move and His brain to function.

Jesus Christ, who'd been dead on Friday night, was quite alive on Sunday morning!

With that, the problem of treason was solved. The Number One Citizen of heaven had taken the place of all the treasonous rebels of earth. Because Jesus is God and infinite, He has the power to take that penalty for each and every one who comes to Him without ever exhausting the supply of forgiveness and payment. All you have to do is renounce your self-will and confess your sins as a result of wanting to be the small-g god of your life. In exchange, as you give back the power you wrested from God, you now have an open door to a relationship with Him in that house called Jesus, forever protected from the lightning of God's rightful wrath for the penalty of every sin you committed or ever will commit.

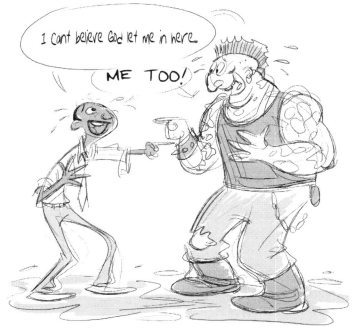

When Jesus died as a man and was resurrected from the dead, the most fearful law known to man—the law of death— was broken. Not only that, God showed that since He has the power to raise anyone from the dead, He can pay the penalty for their treason and give them what He had with them in the beginning, communion with Him, according to His rules.

Forgiveness. Salvation. A right relationship with God? It's entirely God's own doing. That's God's Love, not giving us our way but *paying the debt He was owed in a way that would satisfy His ledger*—and all at no cost to anyone who would humble themselves to ask for it. Not patting us on the head and saying, "There, there, I'll accept your halfhearted measures, and theirs— even if they conflict. Just keep being good enough." There aren't enough good deeds on this planet, not enough energy in your lifetime, to satisfy the eternal debt of treason represented by insulting the One who's infinitely amazing, so God doesn't ask you to even try.

For the nonbeliever and believer alike, this isn't just good news; it's GREAT news.

## Barkeep! Good News for Everyone!

For the nonbeliever—the agnostic, atheist, all-around good person, or maybe some person in another religion trying to do enough good works to appease his or her angry god, the good news is that you have the chance to be forgiven and protected because Jesus paid your entire debt against God for you. All the wrong you've ever done or will ever do won't be counted against you because someone who has the resources to pay for it reached into His deep pocket of grace and paid off your debt. Imagine that in your secret heart! The notion that Someone has shown they love you in spite of all your failings... really? Could anything be better?

For the believer, it's the same and more. Not only are we forgiven and loved in spite of the failings of our rebellion, we have the hope of God changing those flaws in a lasting way that goes beyond their external consequences. If God can raise Jesus from the dead, what can't He change in us? If He's that committed to finding a solution to bring every man, woman and child back into relationship with Him, how much more will He be committed to us once He's saved us as He guides us to cast off the bad habits that cling to us like the stench of cigarette smoke from a French bar. (It's only a bad cliché if you haven't been to Paris and pulled out your coat from the closet six months later and it still makes you gag.) We're forever fighting the desire to scoot off the path in one way or the other, so we're given free access to the Guide and Power that keeps us hiking the one direction to get us home. This gives us hope. Because on the other side of the cross— after you're forgiven, after you learn that God not only forgave you but completely obliterated His penalty for those sins committed, when you've passed from darkness to light— sometimes you have the temptation to think, *Oh great, I have this forgiveness and love, now what do I have to do to keep it going?* The answer is NOTHING. A big. Fat. ZERO. It's a gift! The realization of that gift should forever inspire in us hearts of joy, gratitude and humility as we remind ourselves to look at God who did all the heavy lifting. Yay for the goodness of the gospel!

# But Wait, There's More

In my study about the gospel I discovered that during the course of His ministry, Jesus Himself gave a broader understanding of the good news beyond man's salvation gained through the life, death and final resurrection of Jesus Christ. Instead of stopping there, the Bible says Jesus also spoke about the actual kingdom of God as part of the gospel message (Matt. 4:23; 9:35; 24:14). Jesus, being God, was the only One who was equipped to speak about the subject because, well, He'd been there. He knew God the Father didn't exist in some random, airless vacuum. He'd seen His kingdom home. In thinking about that, it occurred to me that telling anyone only about the death and resurrection of Christ is like giving a foreigner directions to an amusement park without actually helping them understand the amusement park exists. Don't get me wrong, Jesus' death pays the admission price—but just what, exactly, does the price of His shed blood grant the ticket holder?

Residence in heaven, in God's perfect, beautiful and eternal kingdom filled with the light that emanates from Him. A place where there'll be no more tears of pain or struggles from our flawed characters, and where people will live in harmony with one another. Most important, it's a place where the saved of humanity will finally be able to be in the presence of God gratefully worshipping Him for who He is and what He's done.

The gospel that Jesus so often preached is the good news that there's a world beyond this one (Rev. 21). The kingdom He encouraged His listeners to seek wasn't merely a place with streets of alabaster and gold; that's just the location. Jesus presented the goal of the gospel: *to find one's rest at home with God in his kingdom*. One day God's kingdom will swallow this broken and flawed world in blink of an eye. All the houses, cars, and sports games; all the cotton candy, and nightclubs; the jobs we hate, the jobs we love; the blue, blue sky and the birds in it. The pain, the struggle, the joy, the awards, the love and hatred, the striving, yearning, living growing, the wisdom of man and the foolishness in it: all of it gone.

Poof! Just like that.

This world will be changed like a garment and there's nothing we can do to stop it— but why would we? We're not heading to a place of boredom where everyone will be sitting around, strumming harps on puffy clouds, in a food coma after the big marriage feast of the Lamb, for all eternity. We're destined for a kingdom that's the perfect reflection of the God who lives in it. To get a glimpse of the bliss of God's eternal kingdom take look at all of Jesus' commands for how we're to treat one another and comport ourselves before God; then imagine everyone doing those commands joyfully and you'll begin to understand the bliss to be revealed in the kingdom of God.

God who lives in that heavenly kingdom wants to have us in it. However, the only way to enter it is by letting go of everything that belongs to this world, the things that God hates because they offend His character the way the rank smell from that forgotten Tupperware in the back of the fridge makes you gag. God cleans us with the only solvent that can remove the reek of those sins—the shed blood of Jesus Christ.

In the end, the gospel is more than Christ's death and resurrection. The gospel is a restoration with God Himself. So often, though, we forget the joy of that revelation: He's the end. We need to remind ourselves constantly of that hope, in a world that seems more real at times than the reality of God in His kingdom.

That's why I insist that if you don't surrender to the gospel of God, then anything else I say in this book is a like a bag of cotton candy: pretty and fun, but in the end nutritionally empty. In Hebrews 12:2, it's said of Jesus that for the joy set before Him, He endured the cross, despising the shame, and sat down at the right hand of the throne of God. What was that joy? Being with God, His Father, in His kingdom. You too will find joy in the midst of your suffering if you have the hope found in the good news of Jesus. Because not only does believing and accepting the gospel give you the endurance to make it through the upward switchbacks of this life, believing the gospel means God has given you a gift: supernatural power to battle your sinful shortcomings as you anticipate your home in the kingdom of God.

## Ready to be Schooled

Anticipation goes a long, long way!

When I was a little kid, my favorite times of the year were the days just before school started. There was so much hope, as I thought of the new kids and teachers I'd meet and the chance I'd get to see old friends I hadn't seen all summer. I couldn't wait! That anticipation built as I was fitted with new clothes and school supplies the weekend before school started. I wasn't in school yet— but it was the earnest of school to come. I'd spend that night before school started arranging the pencils and pens in the little plastic sleeve, this way and that. Figuring out the best way to put the paper in the binder with the tabbed manila card stock between the sheets. That first outfit— what to wear? Was it that pair of pants and this top? Or was it this collared shirt or that T-shirt? I know it's weird, but I was one of those kids who liked school (well most of it; math and I are still not to this day on speaking terms); the anticipation of it gave me the power to do what was necessary just because I was going to be in school. That I was going to school was a given, because as an American it was my given right, so I didn't work to get to school. Instead *I worked because I was going to* school— and it was my joy!

My joy for school is an analogy: When we believe the gospel that tells us there's a world that will replace this one, in which some of our friends will live, along with new people and ineffable experiences, the life we live now becomes the weekend before the start of school. God's commands are the outfits and school supplies we gather and use in anticipation of going there. If you don't know there's a school, you may get the books, the shoes, and the clothes . . . but in the end, what is it all for? You can use the tools of God to be a better person. You can choose to not steal, lie, commit adultery, or be a glutton . . . for a time. But what happens after that "for a time?" No matter how good you are in this life, you will still have to give an account for the infinite debt you owe God when "school starts" and you stand before Him. There you'll be in anxious anticipation about a test for which you know you've not only underperformed but failed.

It doesn't have to be that way.

You can have an A before you've taken the first class. How? Because Jesus took the test already and passed it for you. Come to Him and ask Him for His forgiveness and salvation then you will have the encouragement to persevere in anticipation of the kingdom to come.

To the nonbeliever, if you don't accept God's invitation to believe in the gospel as written in this chapter, then anything I have to say to you in the rest of pages of this book may help, but there'll be no joy in doing it, no grace when you fail at it and most of all, no hope that, in the end, it'll ever be enough. To you, this book will be another one of those self-help diet pep talks that'll get you excited for a little while, but when the novelty wears off, you'll think I'm a legalist. Or worse, because I brought Him up, you'll blame God for your inability to finish the job.

Look, I don't want that for you . . .

It's hard enough just to live life, let alone attempt to find wisdom and power to deal with the underlying reasons you got fat in the first place. You don't have to deal with your setbacks and trials and just plain "life happens" stuff all alone. If you've read this chapter and desire to have the relationship with God I've described, it can be the easiest decision for change you'll ever make. God is standing ready to receive you, arms wide.

Really, seriously, the God of the universe *is waiting for you* . . . (2 Peter 3:9).

In the book of Acts (chapter 16, verses 30–34), when faced with the mercy of God, a jailer asks a prisoner, the apostle Paul, "What must I do to be saved?" and Paul replies "believe in the Lord Jesus . . ." It's as simple as that. So if you want more than just drudgery—if you want love, a love from God that will lead you to true change— believe in the Lord Jesus and all He's done for you by taking your place on the cross. Believe in the Lord Jesus who was raised from the dead and you will be saved this instant and you will be ready to follow God in preparation for His eternal kingdom. Then the rest of this book will be cake.

But not the fattening kind.

To those who already believe the gospel, in your struggle along the mountain trail toward progressive obedience you'll find joy not merely because of the results, but encouragement because your obedience is the proof of your faith. Also when you fail, as we all do because of our weakness and forgetfulness, you'll find grace to get up and continue, knowing you have a heavenly Father who paid the ultimate price for you to be able to make it to the summit of His love.

If you're a believer, be it newly minted or one who's been in God's family for some time, this book will guide you along the slow and steady path that God brought me on to lose the weight. Eventually you'll find more than less of you as you look in the mirror, you'll find more of a relationship with God as you look into His love.

To finish the story of my friend's conked-out car: We were rescued from the side of the road by someone else in our caravan. Together we made it to Zion. In life there may be second chances, but after we die, God will take into account what gave us power in our daily lives. Was it the power He provides through the gospel or did we try and sneak in on our own steam? As I said, the promise of the gospel is that we will have a relationship with Him. What a shame to make it in your own strength all the way to standing before Him, only to hear him say, "Depart from me, I never knew you."

· · · · · · · ·

Believing the gospel is one thing, but what really matters is how it makes a difference in your life. Faith isn't true faith if it doesn't change how you live. While growth happens at different paces in each believer, transformation *does* happen as God provides supernatural power to effect our natural transformation. The word for it is called regeneration, and I'll address how it looks in a believer's life in the next chapter as I share how God changed my heart to believe in Him and then eventually come to the place where that belief changed my life.

> *He came to His own, and those who were His own did not receive Him. But as many as received Him, to them He gave the right to become children of God, even to those who believe in His name, who were born, not of blood nor of the will of the flesh nor of the will of man, but of God.   John 1:11–13*

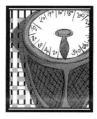

# Take A-Weigh

- Jesus died for our rejection of God saving us from hell and granting us entrance into heaven.
- Heaven is a real place where we will have a relationship with God.
- Believe the gospel and you will have the power and grace to change.

# Food for Thought

*"O taste and see that the LORD is good; How blessed is the man who takes refuge in Him!"*
*Psalms 34:8*

Don't just take my word on anything. Turn to the trustworthy word of God! In the book of Romans, God lovingly provides all who read its pages both the diagnosis for their deadly sin and the cure! Take a walk down the Romans road. Its one stroll that will leave you rested instead of worn out.

*Romans 3:10*
**"There is none righteous, not even one."**

*Romans 3:23*
**". . . for all have sinned and fall short of the glory of God,"**

*Romans 5:8*
**"But God demonstrates His own love toward us, in that while we were yet sinners, Christ died for us."**

*Romans 6:23*
**"For the wages of sin is death, but the free gift of God is eternal life in Christ Jesus our Lord."**

*Romans 10:9*
**". . . that if you confess with your mouth Jesus *as* Lord, and believe in your heart that God raised Him from the dead, you will be saved..."**

*Romans 10:13*
**". . . for 'Whoever will call on the name of the Lord will be saved.' "**

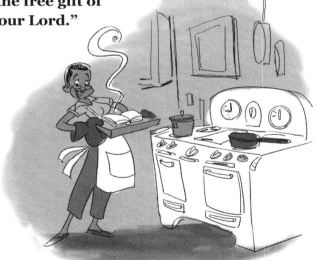

BECAUSE no one ever gained a pound from thinking too much.

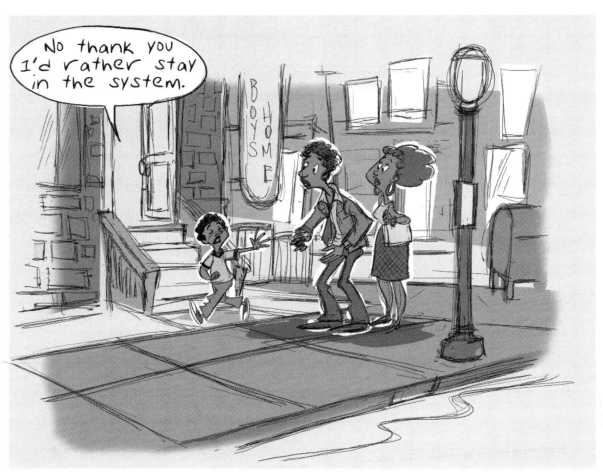

Said NO FOSTER kid to loving parents EVER.

Chapter 2

# The Magic of Regeneration

> *But when the kindness of God our Savior and His love for mankind appeared, He saved us, not on the basis of deeds which we have done in righteousness, but according to His mercy, by the washing of regeneration and renewing by the Holy Spirit, whom He poured out upon us richly through Jesus Christ our Savior, so that being justified by His grace we would be made heirs according to the hope of eternal life.* Titus 3:4–7

Merriam Webster defines the word theology as "The study of religious faith, practice, and experience; especially: the study of God and of God's relation to the world . . ." [1]

Some understandings about God and how He relates to the world are easier to see than others. Other bits of theology are more of the under-the-hood kind. They're like a tiny bolt in the car's engine. It's there, not making its existence readily known: but you won't make it very far if you don't have it.

I'm not a theologian; I'm just someone who gets paid to draw cartoons all day. Thankfully God continues His transformative work in me regardless of whether or not I know the correct words to describe how He does it. I'm glad and humbled He's such a patient God who over time helps me understand why He accomplishes the things in me He does in a way that's unique to me . . . Now my hope is I can explain in a way that encourages and helps you understand how He enables His children to accomplish the things He commands them to perform. The aim of this chapter is to share how the gospel's effect on my life led me to lose my weight, but before I get to that, I want to lift the hood of this car called Christianity and point out one of the bolts that holds this baby together and continually helps me to be *willing* to be willing to change in the first place.

---

[1] From Merriam-Webster's Collegiate® Dictionary, 11th Edition ©2015, Merriam-Webster, Inc. (www.Merriam-Webster.com).

# Restoring the Rottenness

We live in a time where people are preoccupied with zombies. Maybe it's the idea of their unrelenting unstoppableness. Maybe its frustration within ourselves that there's something bad in us we can't overcome. (Sadly, once someone has been infected, there's no hope to reverse the process except really killing an undead person once and for all.[2]) We don't have to prepare for the zombie apocalypse because it's happening now: the Bible says the world is populated with spiritual zombies (Eph. 2:1–2), yet as I wrote in chapter 1, God found a way to reverse the curse by the death and resurrection of His Son, Jesus. However, a person who suffers the effects of spiritual decomposition needs to have the rotten things in them restored.

Restoring the rottenness is called *regeneration*.

Regeneration is the supernatural work of God that causes a spiritually dead person to believe and understand the things of God. When He saves a person, He gives them the spiritual capacity to understand and believe in the Bible and to act on that belief. For me as an artist who was raised on Saturday morning monster movies, just freethinking about regeneration brings to mind some kind of Frankenstein monster sewn together from other bits of dead bodies and electrified into some hulking lumbering mass of misunderstood flesh. It's almost as though God were a Holy Dr. Frankenstein, who brought a dead body back to life. I say almost and here's why: God isn't a mad scientist. He's a loving Father.

Studying the word regeneration as it appears in the Bible conveys a more tender meaning than my monster thoughts, because it means *a new birth*.

How awesome is that? We're not God's monsters, but God's babies. What a loving transformation. Before we were saved, our father was the Devil (John 8:44)—who's a monster, indeed. After God adopted us, we became His children—His babies (Eph. 1:5).

Awww . . . Goo . . .

Who doesn't like babies? Tiny humans whose only defense is their cuteness? They're reliant on bigger humans to care for them, protect and teach them. When God elects to save a person through the gospel, He doesn't just shock them into numb, fumbling, ugly life like some kind of misunderstood monster and leave them to their own devices. No, He tenderly brings them into life like a tiny child with all the patience, nurture and guidance afforded to a tiny uninformed human—all in the blink of an eye.

I'm awed by the magic of regeneration. I know the word "magic" makes it seem fictional. Like a man in a tuxedo pulling a rabbit out of a hat, or a fairy godmother turning a pumpkin

---

[2] I'm sorry for anyone who's offended by zombies. As long as I've been a believer, Romans 8:6–13 has always conjured that image. It's good to understand, especially for those of us who had tamer lives before we believed the good news. We haven't merely been saved from our sins. We were separated from God by our very nature; we were spiritually dead. And like zombies, dead things stink, are self- serving, and are thoughtlessly destructive.

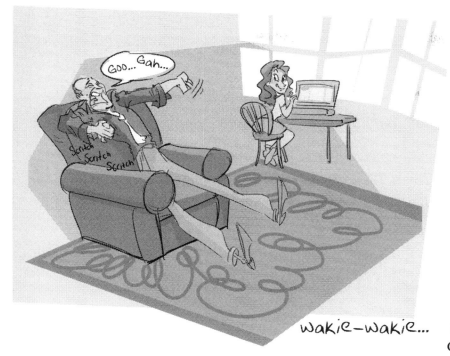

into a coach, but there's something of the child in me that makes me see it that way. God did something amazing when He changed my heart. He put in something that was never there before He acted. There are some who'd say the Bible defines a person's salvation and sanctification (a big fancy Bible word for God's progressive changing a person to be ready for heaven) as not magical, but rather miraculous, but either way don't let my choice of word throw you. Regeneration should fill you with childlike wonder. Why?

Because a Christian's heart is completely transformed by the power of God in an instant.

Once He does this, God sets about helping us understand and eliminate the refuse in our lives that has long obscured the unique people He designed us to be. Some changes in our lives resulting from regeneration become physically visible, while other changes blossom over time in our character. It's a source of great encouragement: God promises that anyone He has saved, He will transform (1 Thess. 5:23–24). However, I know a lot of times, I drag my feet when it comes to dealing with the areas in my life He wants to work with me to clear. Why is this? Often times I justify my faults and actions because I have an emotional attachment to them or because I'm more comfortable staying the way I am rather than go through the hard work of dealing with my sin. I'm sure I'm not alone in this, am I? Thankfully God is more powerful than our reticence to work.

Over the time I've been successful at losing the weight and being disciplined, I've had brothers and sisters in the Lord ask me how I've done it. When I've told them what I will lay out for you in the course of this book, their reply is often a dejected, "Wow . . . I could never do that; I don't have that kind of willpower." You know what, I don't either. That's why I'm glad for God's regeneration in my life, it's what got me going, It's what reminds me Whose I am when I fail, and because of it, I continue to grow and change through obedience to God's Word. Regeneration gives you and me all the power we need to understand and believe God's commands, though it may take some time before we're willing to actually *obey* what we believe.

Regeneration reveals itself in our lives as we listen to and follow God's commands. People can't believe the message of the gospel unless they've first been regenerated. Understanding God's supernatural change that brought you to salvation breaks down the wall between willpower and acting in faith. Because if you believe God's Word when He says He raised Jesus from the dead, (which is an impossible feat) and believe God forgave and paid for your sins, then you have the power to believe that all of His words and commands revealed in the Bible must be the same kind of true. The issue isn't having the power to change, it's that we need to grow in our belief. The point is that we often stifle God's regenerative work in our lives because we make a choice to do it.

Sigh . . . How often I do that . . .

However, the same God who knew how to save you and me also knows how to transform us, and He knows how to strengthen other areas in our character until we're able to obey Him in the areas we once chose to rebel. So let's just stop saying we *can't* obey Him. The moment you acknowledge you have chosen not to obey Him is the moment God can really work. More on belief and obedience in the next chapter.

This is both encouraging and discouraging at the same time. Encouraging because we have the power to overcome any sin God commands us to address, discouraging because the only person who's stopping us from doing it is ourselves. Take hope in this realization: God doesn't leave us alone to fight the battle. While we know the enemy, for it is us, God who knows our thoughts and sees our future knows us even better. Prayerfully ask for His help to fight the war against your flesh and together you'll vanquish your enemy desires.

So understand you have the ability to do everything God's word tells you to do. If you don't, then you're not saved. You can't be powerless in your spiritual life and be connected to the power source found in God at the same time (Eph. 1:18–22). Through regeneration, Christians have the ability to agree with God when He says throughout the Bible that we'd live a lot better without stubbing our spiritual toes on our sinful "stuff," even if it means giving up that treasured behavioral thingamahoozit. Thank God for His grace because your regeneration is your proof of His salvation. Take comfort in the realization that regeneration isn't just having the desire to get rid of the dead acts, its being able to see that finding peace in this world is not the endgame, but it is being with God now and forever. The fact that we consider a relationship with God, whom we can't see, as better than whatever we love here in this life is really pretty wondrously magical, don't you think?

# Finding the Awesome in God's Magic Act

I have a friend who's a professional, close-up magician. He often performs at a special room at the Magic Castle in Hollywood. He's truly astounding. The first time I saw him do some sleight of hand at a friend's Passover Seder, I jokingly shrieked, "Witch, Witch!" While in truth I know my friend isn't in league with the Devil, I can't help but being awed by his abilities that seem to make the impossible possible. Even more astounding, though, is regeneration, because while pulling a card from behind someone's ear is an illusion pulled off by practice and dexterity, regeneration is only accomplished when the dead get brought to life.

*Boom! Try pulling "saw THAT lady in half" for reals and putting her back together and see where it gets you. Hmmmm . . .*

Yet I think today we in the church take the results of regeneration for granted. I think if we had more a sense of wonder at God's act in our salvation, we'd find access to the power to obey God in what He commands.

In the close-up room of heaven, the Bible says in fact that the angels rejoice when someone gets saved (Luke 15:10). They do this not only because God regenerates the dead into life, they praise God because in His regeneration God shows His mercy to a rebellious and dead person. Ponder that in your understanding of God's regeneration: He's done it in love despite the fact that the person He's regenerated was His enemy. If it were up to us we wouldn't regenerate our enemies, we'd squish them. But God isn't like us.

If He spoke all humanity into existence, then really it doesn't take that much effort for Him to say one word and it would be lights out for all of us. God doesn't have to save anyone. He could destroy mankind in a thought. How horrific, all those souls . . . finding themselves not vanished, but vanquished in the torments of eternal hell.

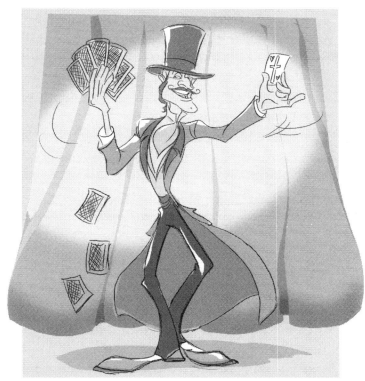

WAS YOUR Card—THE KING OF HEARTS!!!

Look at the world and the state it's in, God could just. Start. Over. No one could blame Him.

So the angels rejoice because God still saves people instead of starting over with a new batch in spite of every sin that every human in every land on the face of the earth has, or ever will commit against Him.

There're as many ways God shows His mercy to people as there are saved people on the planet, so every testimony is a precious reminder of His compassion. Ask your friends to tell you their story of His love, and if they say, "Oh it's not such a big deal; I was never super bad . . ."

or "I didn't get into that much trouble. . . ," remind them that it's not the depth of their depravity they're recounting, but the height of God's mercy they're praising.

**It's your turn—time to stop, put down this book and pick up a pencil . . . or pen, or computer keyboard, whatever is easiest—and write out your testimony. It doesn't have to be perfect. Just spend time pondering what God did for you so that like the angels, you can rejoice!**

If you're a Christian, spend time writing your testimony even though you've done it in the past. I discovered that the testimony I wrote when I first got saved was different than the one I wrote when I started repenting of closely held sin, and the one I wrote several years after walking through the process that became the contents of this book is more nuanced still. It's not that I've remembered different facts, but that God continues to show me how much He has saved and is saving me. Reviewing your salvation story will give you more hope and trust in God's work in your life. So don't be too proud (or lazy) to start over and see how good the Lord was when He saved you.

If you're *not* a Christian, write yours out too. Talk about what your life is like on your own, talk about all your shortcomings and how if you could have the world be any different, how would you like it to be. When I did that, it brought me face to face with how powerless I really was and it wasn't a matter of time before I was crying out to God for His help. Don't be a chicken or prideful and skip this step. Write out your testimony without God: your testimony of yourself.

## Once Upon A Time...

I was saved when I was eighteen. But the circumstances involved in my life since I became a Christian demonstrate God's amazing patience, and His overwhelming love toward me.

As a five-year-old, I had a great aunt who mentioned heaven, and when I said I wanted to go, she told me I was too young to understand. I took her words to heart and dismissed the idea of addressing eternity until I was older. God was calling me then, and though I kept putting Him off, He was always poking at my heart.

As I grew older, I explored doing what I wanted to do in the ways that satisfied me most. Ephesians 5:3–5 says:

> *But immorality or any impurity or greed must not even be named among you, as is proper among saints; and there must be no filthiness and silly talk, or coarse jesting, which are not fitting, but rather giving of thanks. For this you know with certainty, that no immoral or impure person or covetous man, who is an idolater, has an inheritance in the kingdom of Christ and God.*

All of that described my life before God—and I'm mortified to say some of it after I gave my life to Him. In an age where chastity wasn't encouraged, I'm ashamed to think of the things I did, even as a little girl. Each time I brazenly participated in those sins, the pleasure in them was tinged with a hint of dread. Even though I believed in God (but not enough to submit to Him), somehow I knew in the back of my heart He wasn't pleased. Sometimes when the guilt would get too much to bear, I'd try to do good works to pay for the bad feelings.

It never worked. I never found the peace I sought for the wrongs I habitually did.

As guilty as I felt, I still didn't want God to rule my life; He wanted too much. As a child I'd visited a church where the pastor told his congregation that Christ's call to follow Him was total surrender of everything. Even at the age of nine, I didn't want to do that.

During a time when people stepped down from "If it feels good, do it," to "If it feels good do it—but *if you don't want to do it with me then you need to shut up about it!*" God's people were galvanized to get the gospel out there by any means possible. In my teen years, I had many gospel tracts stuffed into my hands on buses by strangers, or I found comic books that talked about Jesus. In the end though, God got my attention in a completely unexpected way.

*The Omen* was released in theaters. The movie is a fictional story about an unwitting family that tries to kill their child after they discover he's the Antichrist born to take over the world. Strangely this story, combined with a comic book I found about the rapture of the church,[3] left me terrified and seriously considering what would happen to me eternally. My mom was a nominal Christian and told me there was nothing to be afraid of: she suggested I just read the book of Revelation to see how the story ends.[4]

For a non-Christian, the book of Revelation is anything but comforting.

So I dragged my mom to church where, after attending a few times and hearing several feel-good sermons about the awesome things God was going to do for me after I died, I walked the aisle and said the sinner's prayer so I could go to the heaven my great-aunt had mentioned and not risk the judgment I'd seen in the Bible. Tra-la-lah. Now I was in good with God: He was my sugar daddy, my grandpa, and my bank. I was assured that one day I'd walk on streets of gold and have a mansion with a big car.

Not surprisingly, though, nothing in my life changed, because I wasn't saved.

The term Christian was coined to describe a person who's a "little Christ" and I was no little Christ . . . I was a big Carole.

So there I was—a vulgar, bawdy, boisterous, sexually immoral, gluttonous hater of God,

---

[3] For those who don't know what the rapture is: It refers to the end times, when God takes Christians from the earth just prior to judging all those who've rejected Him.

[4] The book of Revelation is about when God returns to set up His eternal kingdom. It details a whole lot of plagues and wars. Then after seven years of anguish and terror, all who have refused to bow before Him are judged and cast into the lake of fire.

and though I had plenty of friends, I couldn't shake the fear God was angry with me and my life was in danger.

By the end of my first year in college when I wasn't doing well in my courses as a theater arts major, I came to a place where I realized I needed to take drastic measures. I literally said the words: "I'll do whatever I have to do to succeed . . . I'll even sell my soul to the devil if I have to."

After that, I became afraid all the time . . .

When I was a child I wanted to know about heaven. But before I could understand it, God had to show me the fear of hell. There wasn't anything I could do to shake the dread. Sure I had my friends, but my life was falling apart around me. Due to some personal issues, my family was in shambles, my career future seemed threatened, and now I felt like I was going to die. Looking back now I believe God was gracious to let me feel the full weight of my impending judgment, which preacher Jonathan Edwards aptly described in his famous sermon, "Sinners in the Hands of an Angry God":

> *You have offended him infinitely more than ever a stubborn rebel did his prince: and yet 'tis nothing but his hand that holds you from falling into the fire every moment; 'tis to be ascribed to nothing else, that you did not go to hell the last night; that you was suffered to awake again in this world, after you closed your eyes to sleep: and there is no other reason to be given why you have not dropped into hell since you arose in the morning, but that God's hand has held you up . . .* [5]

In God's providence, that was one of those summers when forest fires were everywhere and the air was black and was filled with the acrid stench of flaming destruction. I was terrified.

Yet into this turmoil and fear of my life came the singular loving voice of God. I worked at a theme park painting airbrush t-shirts. Because I was the assistant manager, I'd open the shop, waiting at Cash Control to get the cash register money for the day. There was another young woman who waited with me some mornings. She was an upperclassman from my school. She was very sweet; little huggy for me—I wasn't used to that—but there was something winsome about her. We'd speak from time to time about acting. She was someone I admired as a talented and beautiful performer. One morning as we waited on the back lot while the sleepy park lurched into activity for the day, she and I spoke about God. I can't remember what she said in its entirety but what words I do remember were:

"Carole, the Bible isn't a book of don'ts; it's a book of dos."

---

[5] *Works of Jonathan Edwards Online,* Sermons and Discourses, 1739-1742 (WJE Online, Vol. 22) (Jonathan Edwards Center at Yale University, 2008), 411–412. "Sinners in the Hands of an Angry God," sermon on Deuteronomy 32:35 (Jan. 1733), (accessed May 7, 2015).

In that simple statement God showed me that He wasn't an ogre. He wasn't standing in heaven with a finger poised to squash me. Instead He had His arms open to welcome me.

My classmate went back home for the summer and I kept working at the airbrush shop, where this new kid showed up: a freckled-faced, redheaded young man with a floppy haircut and a wispy mustache. He was different than the other people in the shop who were a bunch of grumbling prima donnas who picked and chose when or if they wanted to work based on how it benefited them. Being an assistant manager of a bunch of artists was pretty much like herding cats. So by time this kid showed up, I was the picture of the 1 Peter 2:18–20 unreasonable boss and the new kid was the picture of a model employee. He took my every demanding, demeaning request, did work that wasn't his own (losing out on commissions because of it), and he was always on time. In spite of my harshness, for some reason, we became unlikely friends. Eventually I found out he was a Christian and I retreated because I was afraid he would judge me for my life though he never had before I found out he was a believer. So I stood off and I watched him deal with grace as his girlfriend dumped him. I watched him be a good employee. I watched him. And though he never said anything about the gospel, his life was the gospel. So when one day he was late back from break, I was concerned, because as I said, he was never late.

I went to the break room to find him , sitting straight up, his back against the wall. In one hand he held a Coke can, in the other his lunch bag, crumpled in his clenched fist. The weird thing was, he was sitting there with his eyes half closed and his irises rolled back behind his fluttering eyelids. He was trying to not fall asleep. But to me who was terrified of being unprepared for Christ's return, I thought, "Gasp—he's gotten raptured!"

He woke up and went back to work. That Sunday I fled to the little Baptist church where I'd said nine years before I wasn't ready to give up everything and follow Christ.

The pastor's teaching that morning was simple. He spoke from Mark (5:1–20) about the man who was alone, naked among the tombs and was possessed by a legion of demons. The pastor said, "That man was divided and Christ brought him together. Likewise, there are people here who are divided and Jesus wants to bring you together." There it was again—the love of God calling me. Not His judgment, for God in His graciousness was calling me OUT of the judgment that I didn't know I would one day face (John 3:17–18). I had no demons— at least not the literal spiritual kind—*but I was divided.* I knew the person I was in my heart, the scared one vs. the person I was on the outside, the boisterously funny but manipulative one. I wanted peace.

I knew I had to give up everything to stand before Christ but I didn't care, I just wanted to stop being afraid. So I gave God control of my life. I knew I was a sinner, that Jesus died for my sins, that God raised Him from the dead, and I was willing to do whatever He wanted me to do and say whatever He wanted me to say.

Even though my understanding of what it meant to be a Christian was pretty flimsy back then, my life took a different course. I began to not just read the Bible, but now I understood it. The people I spent my time with changed and surprisingly, my career choice changed as well; I repeatedly approached the dean of animation after I told him God wanted me to be in animation and the dean eventually relented even though he insisted I couldn't draw.

From the beginning of summer to the end of it, my life had turned on its head. When my classmate came back to school the first thing I said to her was "Over the summer I became a Christian!"

So many things changed but the most important area was my proclivity to sin. Really and truly that's the sign of new life.

My mind had changed. I longed to please God and He gave me a loathing for what I had once loved.

Yet there were strongholds . . .

There were battles of the worst kind . . . because they were battles I refused to fight.

As Christians there are sins we hate and we despise and point our fingers at those who do them. We cluck our tongues and shake our heads. We righteously state those are "horrible, horrible sins" and God hates those. Indeed that's true. Yet, to some degree we become like the world when asked why should they get into heaven?

*Well at least I haven't murdered anyone.*

The reality of it is, God died for all sins. Not just the ones we find gross. For to God who's perfect, all sins are gross. Colossians 3:5–7 says:

> *Therefore consider the members of your earthly body as dead to immorality, impurity, passion, evil desire, and greed, which amounts to idolatry. For it is because of these things that the wrath of God will come upon the sons of disobedience, and in them you also once walked, when you were living in them.*

For so many years I was like so many in the church as I thought to myself, "I'd never do any of those grotesque sins" while belonging to the "clean your plate twice club" and secretly sitting down and polishing off two medium pepperoni, black olive and mushroom pizzas after dragging them through Italian dressing without giving it a thought.

I'd done so many battles in the name of God. I'd gone to other countries to proclaim His love, served others and happily worked in the church, but the most important submission was so close to home—the kingdom of self I had yet to conquer.

I loved food.

All kinds and in great amounts. Sure I'd lost weight, only to gain in back again. But weight wasn't the issue. My heart was. I was a covetous glutton. Discontent with what God provided and always wanting more than what was right in front of me.

I was much like John Newton, the writer of the hymn, "Amazing Grace," who still trafficked slaves seven years after he became a Christian and only began to fight against it thirty-two years after his conversion. For me, nearly thirty years had elapsed and I had yet to address the nagging voice in my heart.

It's not like I didn't try to repent—halfheartedly. Whether it was in my own strength or with wrong motives, I worked and worked, but nothing I did seemed to work. I did parts of Bible studies and prayed to change my size, but nothing caught. When I'd fail, I'd think, "Well, it's because I'm not walking in the Spirit" or "God just hasn't answered that prayer yet." Each time I'd try and fail, it'd get harder to try again. Eventually, I found myself waiting to feel like obeying.

For me there were no tears. I couldn't make myself feel *anything* for this sin . . . except frustrated. Not that I couldn't get over it—I confess that I was frustrated because I HAD to get over it.

I loved food that much. It was my comfort, my god, my freedom, my control. As a single person, my time was my own. Rather than cook, I'd hit the local restaurants to order my favorites, barely glancing at the menu. Who needed to do variety when I could simply change the location? If I couldn't make up my mind I'd just order both. There were no leftovers in my fridge, they were all liberally stored in the heaping rolls of fat that shrouded my body like a globby, blubbery pillow suit. At 312 pounds by May 17, 2009, my weight was a mountainous task to even consider attacking. So I wasn't going to.

1 John 3:9 says, *"No one who is born of God practices sin, because His seed abides in him; and he cannot sin because he is born of God."* If practice makes perfect, my growing girth showed my perfection. Would God forgive me for being unwilling to repent? It's a frightening thought to think my unwillingness to repent of the double-double burger and giant fries mentality was something which put me at odds with the God who loved me so much He had slaughtered His very own Son.

The tragically sad thing was, as a believer, I knew the right thing to do and I didn't do it. Furthermore, I didn't feel a twinge of guilt over it at all.

I hate to say it was a really bad health scare that put me on the path to repentance because it seems like such a cliché. I guess the only difference in mine was I didn't ask to be spared the consequences of my actions. I was like the prodigal son who came to his senses after living a riotous life (Luke 15:17–18) when I prayed to God, "I don't ask to be given another chance, I deserve the penalty for my actions. After all, I was disobedient, so anything that happens to me as a result of my lack of self-control is my due. I only ask that if You give me one more month, one more week, one more day, that I live it for Your glory." In the end, my health was fine, but I wasn't going back on my word.

I saw my entire life was out of control; meaning, I was letting my excess appetite in all things control me rather than God. I began to learn that the key to why I'd tried and failed so many times to lose the weight was the fact I focused on the externals. The weight. What I wasn't doing was addressing what caused it.

Being under the control of anything other than God is sin. Anything: including food.

Now there are many THIN people who are just as sinful as I was because they're controlled by their love of food even though their body doesn't show it. Yet my corpulence was a result for me of having *sinned* already; I was being greedy, a glutton, a covetous, ungrateful wretch.

God showed me the only way for me to get out of this quagmire of fat was to backtrack. God's plan was so incredibly simple. As plain as the blubber on my belly that obscured my toes . . . and yet it was as hard to do as moving a mountain, because it involved moving my battling self. His plan was this: Since I grew enormous by eating too much, if I just practiced eating until I was satisfied, then eventually, God willing, the weight would take care of itself.

As I thought through my situation, I realized that though I didn't "feel" all those sad, weepy feelings one thinks they need to begin obeying, it didn't matter. I had everything I needed to obey (Eph. 4:22–24).

Waiting for a feeling that might not ever come wasn't going to get me where I needed to go. I'd decided that I wanted the world to know that I was controlled by God and not by food so I made up my mind—and just started walking in what I already knew.

I knew it was a sin to be greedy. So I just. Stopped.

As I was faithful with the little I already knew, God over time revealed to me more and more things to learn to obey, and those lessons He taught and is teaching me are what I've put in this book. But for my beginning I started here:

1) I believed what God said: *"to obey is better than sacrifice"* (1 Sam. 15:22), so I decided not to diet, but rather to eat normally.

2) I believed what God said in Proverbs 19:2—*"he who hurries his footsteps errs."* So I decided I'd have to be patient for HIM to take off the weight in His time, should He be willing.

3) I believed what God said in Mark 7:18-19—*" 'Do you not understand that whatever goes into the man from outside cannot defile him, because it does not go into his heart, but into his stomach, and is eliminated?' (Thus He declared all foods clean.)"* So I made up my mind that I would lose weight eating anything; there were no "bad" foods.

Those were the three points on which God gave me to focus. Eventually, over time, I came to see that God was teaching me *obedience, patience,* and *gratitude.*

In this denial of my desires in order to obey God I found freedom, because He wasn't asking me to sacrifice eating food that He'd created to taste good, He was telling me to stop eating too much of it. As I submitted to His control, even down to what I put into my mouth, I saw that not only is there a right way to live, but that He who tells me how to live loves me very much. By the end of summer, Robin, a woman who'd mentored me for seven years seeing little change said, "If I didn't know you before, I would believe you just got saved."

Unrepented sin, no matter how small, can do that. It can hide the truth of Whose you are.

Recently I over-seeded my nearly dying lawn. After aerating, fertilizing, top-soiling and watering it for two months, all my neighbors were giving me attagirls for all the hard work that paid off in green dividends. However for all the new green grass there were also loads of weeds that needed to be destroyed. The ones that bothered me most were the broadleaf dandelions—I saw them with their little white Afros popping up in various places dotting my lawn. They got my attention and all of my anger. They made me look bad, springing up seemingly as soon as I mowed them down. However one day as I was mowing my lawn, I noticed something else—the clover, low-growing and multitudinous. I didn't pay as much attention to it. It was there, and I knew that a weed and feed would kill it, but it wasn't embarrassing as the dandelions were. But the thing is, they were weeds too, and they were keeping the lawn from being a lawn of pure grass.

I was asked to give my testimony of how God changed my life so I was able to lose my weight and as I thought about putting it together I was struck by something: how ashamed I was that I was going to have to confess my sins of immorality, while not being ashamed at all about all the times I ordered seconds. But sin is sin. As someone once said, "Would you drink a glass of water with a cup of manure in it? No? Okay, how about a teaspoon of it?"

Until we see our sins, both little and large, the same, we cannot fully experience the great love that the sinful woman had for Christ (Luke 7:36–50) when she wept, kneeling before Him washing his feet with her hair, because she knew just how much she needed His forgiveness.

That's what this book is about: how God was merciful to me, saved me and continues to save me, and how He wants to do the same for you. If He has mercifully regenerated you so that you believe the gospel then you have all you need to conquer the sin that keeps you chunky, as well as every other sin known to man. But first, we have to acknowledge that the sin exists.

*No temptation has overtaken you but such as is common to man; and God is faithful, who will not allow you to be tempted beyond what you are able, but with the temptation will provide the way of escape also, so that you will be able to endure it.  1 Cor. 10:13*

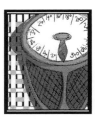

# Take A-Weigh

- Regeneration gives the spiritually dead life and the ability to obey God.
- Every testimony is a wonder of God's mercy.
- God sees all sin the same, so we need to also.
- When we hold on to sins, we can look like we aren't saved.

# Food for Thought

*"But we all, with unveiled face, beholding as in a mirror the glory of the Lord, are being transformed into the same image from glory to glory, just as from the Lord, the Spirit."*
*2 Corinthians 3:19*

I saw a man working in a tree. Actually I didn't see the man, but I could hear him trimming away. Snip. Snip. Snip. Rustle. Shimmy. Drop. Snip. Snip. I took a picture of the tree because it reminded me of how God works in our hearts. Often God's endeavors are not immediately seen externally, but that doesn't mean He's not busily at work. I then saw the arborist's boss, who pointed to three other trees further down the apartment row that had been pruned back hard. "This tree will look like them," he stated with a friendly air of confidence, "but the work has to start inside." From my vantage point I could only see the tree as it was now. Seeing the man's previous good work I trusted this tree would turn out equally well.

I hope you took the time to write your testimony about how God saved you or if you're not saved, how you view God in your life. If you haven't yet, please stop and do it now. Once you're done, fold it up and staple it here on this page. My prayer is that over the course of this book, God will chop away at the hidden tangle of branches in your heart. He'll remove sinful attitudes and misinformed perceptions of who you think He is. You might find that much further along your ideas about God will have taken a new shape even while your body has slowly changed its shape.

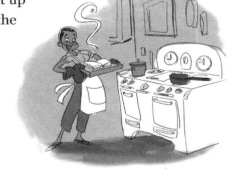

At this point in many weight loss books the author will encourage you to take a "before selfie." This is a good way to record your beginning. I am

Because no one ever gained a pound from thinking too much.

simply asking you to write a spiritual selfie, recording your current understanding of God. You look back on this time and rejoice at the changes He's wrought in your heart. God saved and is saving us. Transformed and is transforming us. While we did start somewhere meeting Him, our understanding of that meeting grows as our understanding of God grows.

Be open to what the infinite almighty God of the universe has in store for your relationship with Him as you commit to tackle this issue. He's not just asking you to learn how to give up your beloved sin. God is helping you make way to make room for Him in your heart. He loves you beyond your wildest understanding!

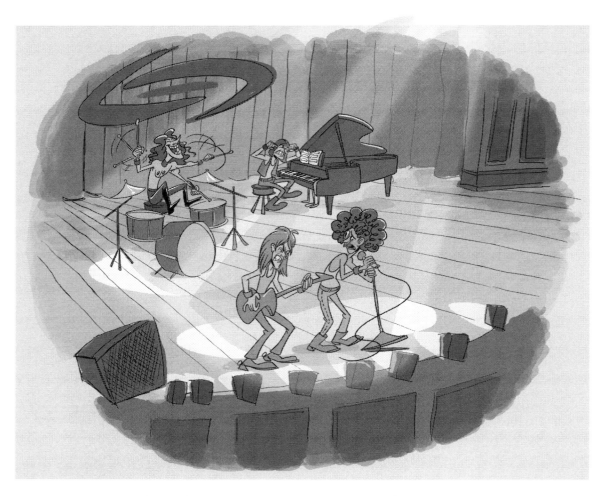

March to the beat of your own drum,
but play the part the way the
composer wrote it.

# Chapter 3

# Wake Up: Time to Obey God

> *My Father is glorified by this, that you bear much fruit, and so prove to be My disciples. Just as the Father has loved Me, I have also loved you; abide in My love. If you keep My commandments, you will abide in My love; just as I have kept My Father's commandments and abide in His love.*
> John 15:8–10

When I was younger I used to have a digital clock radio with the red numbers that glowed in the dark like the beady eyes of some animal. It was set to a local Christian radio channel that broadcasted an early-morning program originating from a large, local Presbyterian church that was helmed by a dynamic pastor with a regal Scottish surname. He was an eloquent man with a bass voice that he used to great effect in his teaching. One week he was preaching a series on obeying God. I remember this because for three days in a row when my clock radio went off in the dark early hour, I seemed to catch the pastor mid-sentence. His voice rumbled and rolled as if it were trying to sound the depths of the Grand Canyon, cutting through my peaceful, innocent slumber with words that rang like a giant, hollow bell:

**"Oh-bey God..."**

It was kind of hard to hit the snooze button on that. I wish I could say the call to greet the day was anything but disquieting. One day I could ignore it. Two days was kind of an odd coincidence. On the third day however, it was laughably frightening. It was as if God Himself had roused me from my bed with loud basso profondo voice, saying, "Get up and do My will today. You've slept long enough."

As quirky as the occurrence was, the topic of obeying God isn't a laughing matter. Jesus said, *"If you love Me, you will keep My commandments"* (John 14:15). Yet often I blithely figure I can take that command to obey His commands as optional.

## Oh, You Want Me to Listen

The Bible translates the word "obey" from the Greek word *hypakoúō,* which means, "to listen" and that listening implies acting on what was said. There are accounts in the Bible

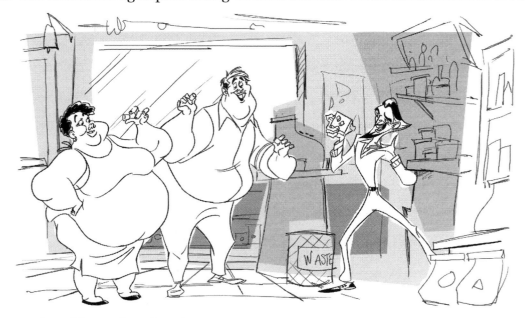

That's right sir and madame. These earplugs are guaranteed to stop ANY unwanted sound. Not even the voice of God can get through these sweet babies!

where Jesus spoke and he was listened to by unlikely sources such as the weather, and demons (Matt. 8:27, Mark 1:27). Just as those things listened to God, we are expected to listen to Him.

Often we choose to be disobedient because God's commands are inconvenient or painful or because we are in pain. Doing what *we* want instead of what *He* wants just feels better. However, the gospel of God says since He forgave and made peace with us, now we're His children and a child is expected to obey regardless of their convenience or feelings.

Interestingly, in the Bible the abnegation of obedience isn't called disobedience, but rather *disbelief.* In Greek, the word that defines this absence of obedience is *apeithéō,* which means, "to not allow oneself to be persuaded, to refuse or withhold belief." While this is an understandable response for nonbelievers to have, it's not acceptable for Christians—at least not for their whole lives.

When we choose to not obey God it's not just that we aren't doing what God told us to do, it's that we are falling into the same trap of disbelief that Eve fell into when she listened to Satan's lies about God in Genesis 3:1-5, namely:

1) God is withholding something good from you.

2) Everything God has given you isn't enough.

3) You won't die as a consequence of your sin.

4) You're smart enough to work everything in your life out on your own.

It's not that we just want to feel better about something in our frustrating or bored or sad situation so we choose not to do what He commands us to do, it's that we think all those incorrect things about God and ourselves so the situation becomes more powerful than Him. Then the *situation rules our life* instead of God who showed His devotion to us when He sacrificed His Son for us.

We need to have a heart of belief that lets us see the reality of God's loving, powerful, protective and all-wise character as stronger than our doubts about how our life appears to be revealing itself at the moment when we're faced with the choice between obedience and disbelief. Therefore if we come to an area in the Bible where we aren't obeying, we need to be like the father in Mark 9:24 who encountered Jesus in his time of need and said, "Lord help my unbelief!"

So when you read the word "obedience" in this chapter and throughout the rest of the book, realize I'm just encouraging you to listen to God and respond in belief.

I'm not saying it's easy. Romans 12:1–2 calls us to be a living sacrifice. A sacrifice in Bible days was put on an altar, where it had its throat slit, or its head pinched off, or was burned up entirely.

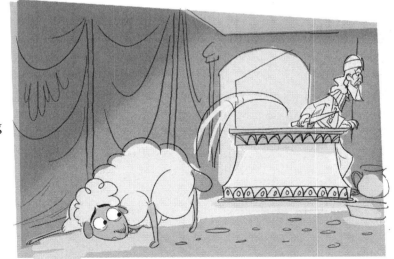

Ahhh . . . good times.

It didn't make the choice to be a sacrifice; someone else made it for them. But when God calls each believer to be a living sacrifice, He's asking us to climb up on the altar ourselves.

Living things have a tendency to attempt to wriggle off the altar when a hand of restraint is removed from them. However God, who has the power to hold us in place and force us to obey, removes His hand and gives us the first lesson in obedience when He says to us, "My first command to you to obey is that you have to choose to do it." He left us the example of Jesus to encourage us to do the hard work of dying to ourselves.

*You mean God wants me to slaughter my will every time I get the opportunity? Come on, He can't know what He's asking. I mean, Jesus had to die only once, but the Father's asking me to do it, well, a lot!*

If you're like me, your reasoning might continue . . .

*God's asking the impossible from me: He's asking me to believe that whatever circumstance is bothering me now on this earth is for His purpose? So instead of choosing to make myself happy by indulging my sinful desires, I need to accept that how God wants me to live in response to this situation is the right way to live? He wants me to be that kind of submitted to His rule over me, not just after I die and stand before Him in heaven, but every minute of every day with every thought and every action as long as I live?!??*

*Ugh...*

If that's what you're thinking, then you, like me, are guilty of being human. I hope by the end of this chapter to encourage you; while hearing we need to obey might elicit a shudder of reluctance, instead it should cause a song of encouragement to break forth from our heart at each opportunity to execute His commands. Why? Because our listening to God's commands proves that His love is in our hearts. Note I didn't say OUR love of God in our hearts, but HIS, because God shows his love to us by calling us to obey because we are His children.

## Stinky Dirty Children

Jesus promised to prepare a place for everyone who believes the message of the gospel (John 14: 2–3).

There's joy in the realization that since we have the promise of a forever place to live, God loves us enough to make sure we get there. That process of getting us there is called *sanctification*. In the Bible, the term sanctify has two meanings: it shows both a Christian's call to be specifically God's as well as a Christian's progressive transformation as we live out our lives. God uses our obedience to His commands to accomplish His sanctification in our lives.

It helps to see the compassion of God in His command for our obedience as not merely because He thinks of us as lowly slaves but because He sees us as His chosen children (Galatians 4:1-7). God loves all His children, even though they have ugly pasts.

Imagine a dark and foul cave full of the worst of creeping things. In the midst of its inhumane conditions, loneliness and exposure scuttle angry, frightened, feral children who long for something better because they've seen glimpses of light, but who have no idea how to reach its source. The darkness is bad, but the things they find in the cave to content themselves make it *almost* livable. Then, in spite of the fact that the wild children are filthy and blinded by living in perpetual darkness, God rescues one into the bright white light of His presence, and He holds the spitting, clawing and kicking feral child tightly to His breast and says, "You are mine . . . "

Now, although the child is no longer an orphan, the cave's rank stench still clings to him, even within the arms of a loving, pure and clean Father, so God scrubs him intently in preparation for his future life in the Lord's eternal, indescribably remarkable heavenly kingdom. In this new home the foundling will no longer live as an untamed beast but now as a royal heir, and everything wondrous he could ever have dreamed of will be right before his eyes for eternity because he'll be with God who's the source of all good and the fulfillment of all humanity's deepest longings. Until move-in day, the adopted heir still has to practice the directions laid out by the Father that will prepare him for his forever home. This does not imply that he must obey in order to *merit* that home, mind you. But since he's now a child of God by His own choosing, he's already destined for it.

On this earth, human beings are the feral boys and girls who scramble and claw through the darkness of this life. In the cave, they mistake the glimpses of God's grace—good food, enjoyment of their bodies, relationships and successful jobs—as all there is to be had; they find satisfaction with whatever they can in their effort to comfort and preserve themselves. They've no idea about the life outside of the cave. God in His mercy and foresight picks each and every single one He calls to be a Christian from the darkness, calls them His own and cleans them up through the washing of His Word in the Bible as He directs them home.

So in essence those are the two forms of sanctification at work: the part where the person is called by God out of darkness, and the part where the person is continually taught to walk in the kingdom of light, navigating their way to live in God's heavenly Kingdom for eternity.

God doesn't just choose people to be supplicants who slavishly worship and grovel before Him for scraps of whatever He feels inclined to dispense that day. No, unbelievably, He makes children out of the very people who'd rather have nothing to do with Him. (John 1:12–13; Rom. 8:14–16; 1 John 3:1–3). Each person God has chosen has this hope, because their heavenly Father is committed to sanctify everyone He's adopted.

In the practice of adoption, people generally want to get babies: the idea being that they don't have to undo a lot of bad programming from bad parenting by other people or other situations an older child might have experienced. This is a sad and difficult reality for older children who find it hard to find adoptive parents, "forever homes." Yet when God adopts an orphan sinner into His home, it's as if He is opening His heart to the worst of the messed-up older children: people who've been scarred by tragic circumstances, lifetimes of foolish choices, and abuse suffered at the hands of other broken "orphan children." What amazing love, patience and kindness He shows in doing this.

The point can be missed if one's just obeying for the straight sake of obeying. The point is—you're adopted! No person who adopts an older child does it out of obligation but chooses to make that child part of their family out of love and compassion. They as parents don't do it because they need something back. Rather they do it because they see the need of the child and know they have an abundance to offer, even if their abundance is nothing but love. God is that adopter. He chooses each of us feral children with the realization we have nothing to offer Him in return and He has everything to give. His home is spotlessly perfect because, well, it's the home of God. Of course there are expectations, so we don't "track mud" of the world into it. When we practice obedience over our lifetime, we learn to look like the Father who loves us.

# Going Home Now . . . Okay Now . . . How About Now?

Long road trips are exhausting. Especially when you're riding in giant black car across the state of Texas with the windows down because your father doesn't want to run the air conditioning, so you have the extra bonus of longhorn steer air freshener for the eons it takes to cross the state. Even though the trip is a trying one, you're still expected to behave like you're part of the family, and not punch your sister if she crosses the invisible line in the back seat. Obedience to God's commands in this life is much the same. We're on a looooong road trip; the destination is our future home (Col. 1:13).

No one who's saved has done anything to merit his or her salvation, God has brought each believer into His holy family by His gracious choice. That being said though, each adopted believer this side of the cross of Christ is called to live in submission to God (Rom. 6:8–14). When we practice submitting to God's commands, we live our lives now as we'll live them in our heavenly home for eternity.

Every country, every hamlet, every home has rules. People indirectly set up the rules (laws) through their elected officials. They all agree to the laws and think they're a pretty nifty thing, for without them, that town would be a horrible place to live—and no one could get through an intersection. So there are rules for traffic, rules for when the garbage cans go out on which night, rules for how loud the music can be and for when workers can start demolition on the neighbor's house. The rules are the boundaries, set up so we can live with each other in harmony. But if we don't follow them—when the neighbor tells his contractor to start at seven instead of eight; when someone blows through the red light because she's running late; when two kids break into your house while you're on vacation— we cry out for justice.

We get this. So with our understanding that rules make for a more harmonious society, we somehow think that there are no rules in heaven?

Heaven is more than just a land where we'll see our long-gone family and get our rewards; it's an actual place. So if we acknowledge that every land has rules, then heaven must have them too. The only difference in heaven's rules is that they're not created by someone we voted in as the lesser of five evils. No, the edicts of heaven are from Someone who's perfect and wasn't voted in because heaven's His home and He knows how He wants it run. The rules of the new home therefore aren't arbitrary, like when your parents got tired of your questions and responded with a sharp, "because I told you so." No, they're actually pretty perfect, awesome rules because they're the mirrors of a pretty perfect, awesome God (2 Cor. 3:18).

When God was leading Israel to the Promised Land He gave them the commandments with the promise, "do this and live." Those rules set the Israelites apart as His own particular people, and the commands were to be obeyed on the way to the Promised Land as well as once the people of Israel were in it. Now for those of us who have been saved by the death of His Son, God says, "do this BECAUSE you live" (2 Cor. 5:17; Eph. 2:10). So if you find you're struggling with the concept of obedience, the ultimate issue is not your problem with obeying—but your understanding of where your home actually is.

I can practically hear people thinking, *Wait, you mean I'm not saved because I can't stop sinning in this area?* Hooooold on a minute there! I can't speak as to whether or not you're sincerely saved—but if you've submitted yourself to the gospel (as I spoke about in the first chapter) then you're saved. So it's not that you can't stop sinning in this area or that area—but that you *won't* stop sinning in this or that area.

You, my friend, are a little lawbreaker. You're breaking the laws of your future home.

Let's pause to remember as believers that "keeping the law" as described in the Old Testament can't save us, because it's weakened by our sinful flesh. Therefore the law isn't powerful enough to pay the penalty for our sins to a God who demands death as the price of our pride (Rom. 8:1–4). So we place our faith in God who paid our debt Himself with the price of His perfect Son, Jesus. God the Father poured all of His righteous wrath, which we rightly deserved, on His Son, who did nothing to deserve that wrath. In doing this, Jesus became the total, final and completely effective substitute payment for all who come to Him for salvation. He removed all eternal condemnation from us for when we humanly fail.

However, that doesn't mean we don't have to be attentive to His commands, everything Christ told us to do, directly in His own words or through His apostles' and follower's writings laid out in the Bible.

This isn't your home. Heaven is.

When you obey God's commands, whatever they may be, you're not merely knuckling under and "doing the right thing," you're actually casting your eyes forward, beyond your picky, petty boss; past the person who cut you off in traffic or the family member who disrespected you or the boyfriend or girlfriend who dumped you. You're looking toward your *real home.* Conversely, when you don't obey God's rules, since you're a citizen of heaven by the death of Jesus Christ—you're quite plainly breaking the law. You're no different than the two men who broke into my neighbor's house and had to be hunted down by twenty cop cars, a helicopter and a K9 unit.

When we sin, we become practical atheists in our disbelief. The problem comes down the fact that we forget during the course of the day as we march across the desert of our lives, our jobs, our relationships and our personal circumstances toward our heavenly home, that GOD has given us commands to prepare us for our eternal rest summed up in Jesus' command of "be holy as I am holy" (1 John 3:4).

Okay. Take a moment and breathe.

Lest you become overburdened with the realization that each decision you make to disobey God makes you a wanton criminal . . .

As I'm writing this and STILL struggling with my appetite, the weight of these words is enough to discourage me.

This is why we always go back to the gospel and Jesus' love for us over and over again. Do you think God would exhibit such patience when you (and I) were rebelling against Him in ignorance before we were saved only to throw up His hands and say, "Ugh, I can't believe they're still doing this! I give up . . . Later, losers," *after* He's given us new life? God's patience is what leads us to repentance so if He gave up on us for all our failings, how patient would that be? No, God's in it for the long haul, whether you're rebellious or not. He, who raised His Son from the dead will exert the same power to both forgive and transform us in our rebellion. So each time you fall, don't give up: instead, get up, ask Him for forgiveness and help and continue on following as He directs you in the Bible.

Thinking on this should cause a believer to erupt into songs of praise and gratitude to Him who forgives each act of rebellion with the same eagerness now as before we were saved when we crawled to Him in contrition and humility and said, "Forgive me, Father for I knew not what I was doing." In truth though we stand condemned by the reality that we're lawbreakers, the greater truth is that God has taken care of the penalty for our treason in His Son (Rom. 6:22-23; 8:3–4).

Treat each act of obedience as the actual goal of your daily life and not a way to get to heaven. We who are saved are already going there. The apostle Paul and the other epistle-writers often addressed the readers of their letters as "saints" not people who "will be saints" (Rom. 1: 7; 1 Cor. 1:2; 2 Cor. 1:1; Eph. 1:1; Phil. 1:1; Col. 1:2). He called them saints because God had already made them so. They didn't have to do anything to get the title. God had already placed them in the Kingdom, so the epistle-writers were just letting them know, "since you are already a saint in the land of the King, this is how you should be living."

Bottom line: Obedience to His commands isn't so we will get to enter heaven but because these are the rules of the home where we are already installed.

The moment you forget this, obedience becomes dry and powerless. I think that's why it says in Hebrews 12:2 that *"for the joy set before Him,"* Christ *"endured the cross, despising the shame."* It wasn't the joy of the cross—that was the obedience part (Phil. 2:8). It was the joy that He was going home to where His Father lives.

The moment you focus on the earthly results—how fast or slow it's going, in the case of the sin that creates long-term weight gain, whether you're looking for people's approval or at how snug or loose your pants fit—then it gets tiring. Given enough failure or not enough applause, you'll eventually give up. If you fall far enough you won't even want to try. Trust me, I've been there.

So now that we know that there are rules for our new home, and that we're to live governed by them as we make our way there, the next question we must ask is, what does obedience look like?

# The Simplicity in Doing

In chapter 9 I will address possible hindrances to carrying out the task of obeying. Now let me encourage you that every little obedient step you take is as if you've taken a giant leap because, as a former spiritual zombie, you're showing God's regenerative life in you! So don't underestimate the importance of doing what God reveals to you to do, no matter how simple it seems.

One day while doing a job at a dear friend's house, I dropped a pencil on the floor. You have to understand, the desk I was working at was like ten feet tall... well, not really, but it sure seemed like it. It was perched on cinderblocks to make it easier to be a standing desk so that anyone who used it seated would have to perch themselves on a chair raised to its full height and then hop that extended chair across the floor to get to the tabletop. From there, the seat-ee's feet dangled from the seat like a six-year-old's in a grown-up restaurant. The process was a royal pain so when the pencil slipped from my hand and fell to the floor, I opted to leave it there and grab one of the *other* pencils at the summit of the desk where I was already. After a few minutes I called my friend to check my work and as she approached me, without her eyes leaving my project, she stooped, caught the pencil in her fingertips, put it back on the tabletop and commented on my drawing. I thought at that moment, *"Oh . . . that's why her house is always so neat."* I realized my friend always had a neat home because she was in the habit of "picking up the pencils" in her life instead of waiting for the avalanche to come. Really simple.

God's commands are that kind of simple. Nowadays I think we make it so much harder than it needs to be. When John the Baptist called people to repent he said to the soldiers, "You stop taking money that's not yours." (Lk 3:14) Zacchaeus said he'd return things that he'd stolen, even if it went as far as far as giving more than what he'd taken. (Lk 19:8) Repentance in those cases was just simply making things right. Sometimes we as Christians don't think "being right" as revealed in God's word is good enough. We pray, look for formulas, memorize verses and do all of these extra things to overcome sin, but we don't actually do the simplest thing, which is just stop sinning in the area God shows us is opposing Him.

Am I saying this simplicity of obeying is easy?

Noooo. In fact it's the hardest thing you'll possibly ever do: because you're turning the control of yourself over to Someone else, so you'll be fighting the pull of your past practices. It's a tough slog at times. We're going to fail. Sometimes we give in to our sinful desires—but when we repent we have the assurance that our Father loves and forgives us (1 John 1:8–9). Of course growth in obedience takes time; it's pretty much lifelong.

## Even Lucifer Believes in Jesus

So often we find ourselves frustrated with our progress in the Lord so we don't do anything. Instead we need to look at obeying God, even in the small things, as the steps that lead to eventual great growth. For example in the case of eating; you might think it's a silly little thing to put down the fork when you've had enough rather than getting more food, but if you do that consistently, you might achieve not only weight loss, but also unexpected growth in other areas of character you thought were impenetrable strongholds.

When I first started down this road of repentance, I acknowledged my ambivalence toward obedience to what the Bible says about how a believer is to approach eating and commitment to God. I prayed. I was going to move forward in what He had revealed regardless of my feelings. I decided that, since I believed that Jesus is God (and no one can do that unless the Father provides the power to do so), I had everything I needed to obey God's commands. In a sense I rolled up my sleeves and said, "God left in the Bible His commands for how I should relate to food. I believe it, and that's enough for me." (These commands will be outlined during the course of this book)

A friend challenged me on my statement that our evidence of belief in Christ was enough to justify our further belief in doing all the things God commanded through His word. "Even demons believe," she said, referring to James 2:19. She made a good point, to which I reply here in the pages of this book that the difference between a demon's belief and a Christian's belief is that the malignant spirit's belief doesn't lead to obedience. If you're a Christian, then you need obey God in what He commands you in order to show evidence of it by moving beyond demon faith, a faith that acknowledges God, yet doesn't do anything He says (James 2:18–24).

Living this way was how I began to bring my appetite into submission. It's also how I'm

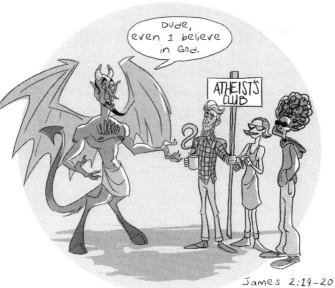

Believe so as to obey.

able to pick up and keep going in the times when I desert Christ and return to my sin (when I allow life on earth to be more real than the reality of heaven).

The glorious bonus of obeying God is that when we do, we see a continual demonstration of God's saving power in us, because each time we choose His way over our former manner of life, we demonstrate the explosion of His life within us. While you can only be saved once, obeying God becomes that salvation in action. I'm tempted, but I'm saved, so I choose to act on what my Savior has commanded, thus demonstrating that He saved me from darkness and gave me the power to believe and act on His commands—and that transforms me.

In the same way that running is actually a series of sustained rapid movements to keep one from falling, obeying God is our spiritual run. As we move from one opportunity to choose God over ourselves to each subsequent choice of obedience, our spiritual run becomes more and more graceful. Even when at times we stumble over our pride and have to repent and return to what we know we ought to be doing, we are reminded: *"The steps of a man are established by the Lord, and He delights in his way. When he falls, he will not be hurled headlong, because the Lord is the One who holds his hand"* (Ps. 37:23–24).

## Not New Lives in Bondo®-ed Wrecks

I grew to appreciate vintage cars after my friend purchased a beat-up old 1961 Studebaker Hawk. Over the next several months he poured time and money into that hulk and turned it from an eyesore to a showpiece. There wasn't one detail he overlooked from the inside to the out; it was fantastic! For all the spit and polish my friend put into his baby that still gets looks from other drivers when he idles next to them at a stoplight, it's nothing to be compared with what God has planned for those who are His own. God doesn't intend on merely tidying our lives to live in heaven, He tidies our lives up so we will live in heaven in new incorruptible bodies for all eternity (1 Cor. 15:37–40). I don't know precisely what that means, but I'm sure the body God gives us won't have a trace of heavenly Bondo®.[6]

---

[6]  Bondo® is autobody filler used to fill dents and dings before a car is painted. The damage remains though hidden by paint.

I think that's the reason God doesn't describe in the Bible what the Christian should look like, size-wise. However, He does spend a great deal of time describing the character of the hidden person of our heart that will reside in His heavenly home. God is more concerned about how we'll live when we join Him in heaven then how we strive to look here on earth. Earthly looks can be deceiving. That's why God sees the mountainously large one the same way He views the stick-thin one that practices the same sins described later in this book. Both of them have the same flaws of character in their heart; it's just that one's sin is more visible. Seeing that God's desire is to transform your heart (His primary goal) should give you patience when your weight loss is slow; remember that God is at work in you creating lasting change beyond these bodies that depreciate with the advance of time.

More on patience and detours later, but the important thing to remember is progressive success in obedience is the more valuable prize, not the smaller dress size.

Therefore, what I outline in this book isn't oriented to get you down to a size six, or zero, or whatever size you believe the fashion magazines tell you should be. The reason for my words is to encourage you to relinquish the control of your life to God in all respects—even down to the amount of food you put in your mouth. The weight loss is actually the fat icing off the top of the cake.

Okay, I hear some of you saying by this point, "Well that's fine for you; you seem to have it down. Look at all that weight you've lost. But I keep failing, so why even bother?" Believe me, I DON'T have it down. This is as much a reminder to me as it is to you. The process of obedience is a gradual one. As I'll say repeatedly, very rarely is anyone poofed into perfection. It takes time.

When I started writing this book, I was up thirty-five pounds from the one hundred and fifty I'd lost because I stopped doing the things I knew were right due to various "feelings." I'm so very thankful for His grace and forgiveness when I fail. What you see is not someone who's perfect, but someone who's being perfected, and it's a long hard race to death's finish line. However, the One who stands at the finish line to give me a ribbon, also stands on the sidelines to cheer me along the way. Not only that, He runs with me to encourage me to keep going.

So to sum it all up, we're called to obey God. Our obedience is just learning to live now on earth the way we will live in heaven. We don't do it because we feel one way or the other about it, but because we're called to do it. It's the encouraging evidence that we're actually saved. Even though we struggle at it, we have a loving Father who's there to forgive our failings and love us all the way home.

Are you awake now? "Oh-bey God!"

· · · · · · ·

*No man shall ever behold the glory of Christ by sight hereafter who does not in some measure behold it here by faith. Grace is a necessary preparation for glory, and faith for sight. Where the subject (the soul) is not previously seasoned with grace and faith, it is not capable of glory or vision. Nay, persons not disposed to it cannot desire it, whatever they pretend; they only deceive their own souls in supposing that they do so. Most men will say with confidence, living and dying, that they desire to be with Christ and to behold His glory; but they can give no reason why they should desire any such thing— only they think this somewhat better than to go to Hell.*

*John Owen*, The Glory of Christ

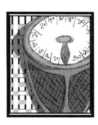

# Take A-Weigh

- Obedience is listening to God.
- Our obedience in this life prepares us for our eternal home.
- Every act of obedience is a great act of God's work.
- Christians demonstrate their belief in God by obeying Him.

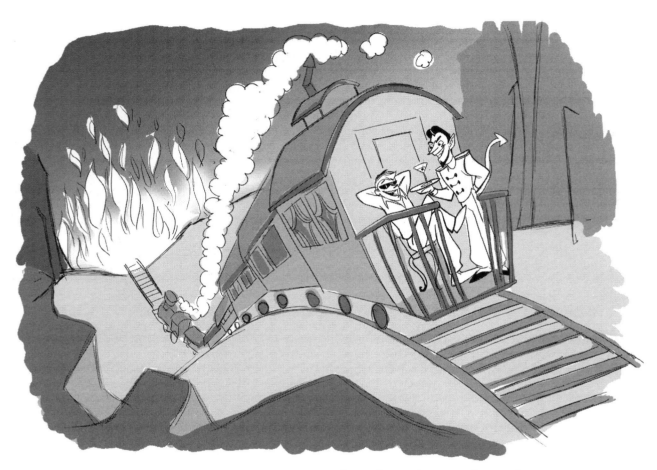

Aaaaahhhhh... This is the life!

# Chapter 4

# The Death Row Dieter

> "When the Pharisee saw it, he was surprised that He had not first ceremonially washed before the meal. But the Lord said to him, "Now you Pharisees clean the outside of the cup and of the platter; but inside of you, you are full of robbery and wickedness. You foolish ones, did not He who made the outside make the inside also?" Luke 11:38–40

If you talk about sin with the average non-Bible believing person, they'll often default to the worst thing they can think of: "Well, I'm not that bad . . . I haven't murdered anyone." Likewise, Christians will justify their "little sins" by saying "I'd never indulge in anything huge like immoral sex."

Murder and sex?

*Seriously that's all there is? Phew, that makes this whole repentance thing easy. Just don't murder anyone and whatever you do, don't participate in any immoral sex act. Ever. Check.*

Humph... Seems like an awful big waste of time and effort for God to become a man, live a sinless life, be killed and raised again from the grave for just the small population of sexually immoral and murderous people of the world, but oh, well.

That is—unless there's more to sin than just those two acts. The fact is there's more at stake than what we see when a person indulges in committing those two acts or any sin on this planet because sin isn't merely a person's acts, sin is a person's inclination of heart (Matt. 15:1–19).

According to both the Old and New Testaments, the heart is the seat of who we are as a person, both physically and spiritually: all our knowledge, memories, inclinations, emotions, passions and appetites are included in what the Bible refers to as our hearts.

God doesn't just save a person and tell them, "Stop doing naughty things." That doesn't work, because the desire to sin still remains in your heart even while you choose to not let it promote the action to do that naughty thing. Instead, God addresses a person's

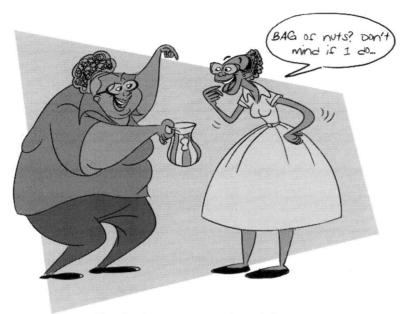

The battle is in my heart not in my buldge.

heart as the source of why he or she does sinful things and gradually changes those desires, which in turn gives that person the power to overcome the acts, not with resentment, but with joy.

Before we can address actions that can make us put on weight or not lose it, we need to first understand internal drive that causes us to sin. I called this chapter "The Death Row Dieter" because it's quite possible to do all the right things to promote change, but still to have a heart that wants to keep on sinning.

As I first mentioned in chapter 1, "Charging the Battery," from the beginning of mankind when God created Adam and Eve, He told them if they ate from a certain tree in the garden they'd die. But they believed the lie of Satan instead of the Word of God and indulged in the fruit of the tree of the knowledge of good and evil. While they didn't die in the strictest sense of keeling over right there in the Garden (full face plant, lights out, game over folks), they died spiritually in their hearts and suffered the consequence of being left to figure out life mostly on their own because they were now separated from God who'd been with them physically, teaching them how to walk in His ways. Eventually Adam and Eve had children who were also spiritually stillborn (Gen. 5:1–3). Their very first son chose to walk in his own way, even though God would counsel that son in the right way to live from God's heavenly home until finally, that spiritually dead son committed an actual physical murder (Gen. 4:1–8).

And so the story continues as humanity continues to make more humans; sin happens and death in some form is its result. It may not be a murder in every case, but all sin creates some kind of deathlike destruction. Eventually the penalty for living as a spiritually dead person is to one day become a real dead person (Rev. 21:8). It's not because God is vindictively lashing out at people and killing them for disobeying Him; it's because people have been born with the inclination to step off the only path that leads to life. They do this willingly, like their first way-back-at-the-beginning-of-time grandparents, without regard to the consequences of their choice.

God's big desire is to restore mankind's relationship with Him, but he doesn't want fakers: people who merely *do the works* but don't mean it. He wants people who genuinely want to be with Him. He's looking for genuineness that comes from the heart. So God, the Master Surgeon, uses His word like a scalpel to cut the cancer of sin from our hearts.

It's understandable to be distrustful of anyone who comes along and says he wants to perform heart surgery on you unless he first points out that there's a consequence to not having the surgery done in the first place. Particularly if you don't feel like you're dying.

## Either the One-Way Street or the Dead-End Road

Think of it this way. Imagine you're hiking on a dark and treacherous path. You've no light but you can't stop walking because, well, who wants to stay on a dark and treacherous path. Someone who claims to know the path comes along and offers you a headlamp to show you the way, and you're all like, "No, I'm good, I think I can figure this out on my own." However what you don't realize is that this dark and treacherous path is eventually going to come to an even darker and more treacherous drop from a cliff that's disguised by a tangle of bracken, which also hides a slender bridge that's the only way across the bottomless ravine to the other side where there's safety and a lovely, warmly lit cottage. So you trudge along, singing a happy song or maybe talking about your favorite sports team, oblivious to the danger you're in. Well, not completely unaware, because the person repeatedly insists you take the light as he says, "There's a cliff ahead on the road with a tiny bridge, if you don't have this light you'll miss it and die!" Even with that warning, you in your pride and with the fact that you can at least feel the ground beneath your feet, believe you'll be okay walking the way you want. You trust that you'll find the path to the cottage by yourself. (Or if you miss it and do die, you'll get put back on the path to try and find it again.)

The point I want to emphasis in this analogy is; there are many ways to fall from the cliff, but only one way to the path of the cottage where God lives. As a person walking in your own way, it's just a matter of time before you topple off the cliff to your doom.

That's what sin is: Walking in your own way. The Bible defines the word for sin as missing the mark or wandering from the law of God. When God directs us to walk in His ways rather than our own, it's not because He's a stuffy killjoy, it's because He's demonstrating that He's a God of peace: a peace that provides harmony with Him as well as unity with one another (1 Cor. 14:33).

Imagine a classroom full of children where everyone's doing what you asked . . .

That is, except for two or three children who aren't being really, really bad, but they are just kind of spinning around or looking here and there, or giggling and in general being mildly distracting.

Eventually it'll spread to the other children until you're standing there shouting at the top of your lungs, "I'm the teacher! I'm the teacher!"

Now imagine an entire world full of those kind of squirrelly children, and God's the only teacher who knows everything. It makes sense to have rules, and it makes sense to shut down the distractions ASAP, or else the world class is in anarchy.

I've made the concept of sin appear the way that most people see it. Not that bad, like disruptively giggling or not keeping one's hands to oneself, but that's just for the point of illustration. God actually sees every sin, no matter how small, as evidence of a bigger problem, which is a sin-sick heart. You can see just how grave this sickness is when you look at the consequences of letting it run rampant in your body.

# A Holy Impact Statement

Sin, according to the Bible, is breaking God's law—and everyone does it (Rom. 3:10–18). We may not all be murderers, fornicators, drunkards or cheat on our taxes, but we all sin in one way or another because our heart longs to do what we want instead of what God wants (Rom. 3:23). In the end, because God is the perfection that identifies what is holiness versus sin, He'll be the Judge who'll inflict the penalty to suit the crime of failing to be the reflection of Him (Eccl. 12:13–14).

In a court of law, victims get to face their attackers and weigh in on the impact of how their crime has forever changed their lives. That way criminals not only receive the penalty of their crimes, they're also left with the actual impact of what their crimes have done to other human beings. Once imprisoned, they're left with time to ponder that.

We think this forced self-reflection is a good thing. Not only because we think criminals will learn something from it, but also because it's just. A piece of you has been forever assaulted. You might learn to work around it, but never again will you be like you were before it happened. It's punishment. You lose, and so do they. They too will be forever changed, even locked up with the key thrown away forever. It seems like a pretty fair shake.

When a person dies and stands before God, it is the *One who created the rules* who gets to deliver the impact statement against those of us who've broken them. Not only does God deliver His impact statement, He also enforces the penalty for the crime. Can you imagine what would happen in the courtroom if the judge was the injured victim who also delivered the verdict?

Shudder.

If a victim were to impose the penalty against the one who committed the crime against him, it might lack compassion and only seek revenge. However God is not like humans. In fact He takes no delight in the death of the wicked (Ezek. 18:21–23). But when a person sins against Him, definite consequences are built in.

The penalty of sin is eternal death—a death where the criminal is left to ponder the awareness of how HUGE the crime of rejecting God is.

Joseph Mengele was nicknamed the Angel of Death in Hitler's Nazi Germany. He was a horrible, horrible person who conducted horrifying experiments on Jewish prisoners because he didn't see them as human. He also determined who went to the gas chamber and who didn't. When the Germans lost the war, he, like a few other Nazi criminals, escaped to Argentina where he lived to a ripe old age, eventually drowning while he was swimming.

*Wait, what? He just drowned as an old man? That ain't right!*

When I heard that in my twenties I was horrified. "This horrible, horrible man never paid his debt for doing those horrible, horrible things, although they tried to get him to return to stand trial?" I sputtered and fumed to my coworkers. I felt that my righteous indignation was justifiable. I wished that they could dig him up, bring him back to life in order to kill him, and then bring him back to life and then kill him again and bring him back to life . . . And as I thought about it, it dawned on me—that's just what hell is.

A constant death. A constant pain. On top of that, an awareness of your wrong, with eternity to pay for it. It doesn't matter if the sin was little or large; it's not the sin that's the measure of the punishment. Rather, the weight of the sin comes from the One who has been sinned against. If the death of six million people cries out for justice, though they were imperfect people themselves, how much more does rebelling against the life of the perfect One God demand justice?

That's why the penalty of sin is so great and eternal, because all have sinned against God who's eternal. It goes beyond a classroom of mildly rowdy kids to a direct attack on the character of the perfect God.

Christ didn't just die so we'd be forgiven for our sin. If the whole earth were forgiven of the acts of rebellion, that still wouldn't be enough, because there's still fruit that has to be reaped. It's as if, thinking we'd planted healthy plants, we have actually sown an orchard of lies, murder, slander, greed, immorality and the like. It's not enough for God to say, "Hey, bro, I forgive you for planting all those nasty trees," and leave it at that. No, something has to be done, because that fruit's coming down sometime, and all of it is deadly (Prov. 14:12).

When Jesus Christ died, He gave us something we couldn't get on our own: God's very own personal righteousness. He paid the penalty for sin; in effect, He harvested all that poisonous fruit so we wouldn't have to. So every rowdy child that comes to Him from the class of earth is given a not just a clean slate, but they're saved from the danger of death. With His power, they're then equipped to see the poisonous trees in their lives and not only cut them down, but dig them up, roots and all.

The disease of sin that sends each and every person to eternal hell is what God is at-tempting to remove with the scalpel of His Son. That's the first step. The next step is to submit to all God commands so we change from the heart.

*When God gave His son to die on the cross, He died on my behalf so that now all I have to do is fight my sin, not pay for it.*

This is why there is no grievous sin (except dying without accepting Jesus Christ). No murder no fornication, no lie that is greater or lesser. It's all against God, so it's all equally bad. God hates sin, not because He hates people but because it's a direct assault on Him (Pss. 50:16–23; 107:10–22).

Just to be clear.

Sin is being anything or doing anything God isn't or doesn't. It's being unlike God.

And if that isn't enough . . .

Sin isn't just the action of doing sinful things—the Bible says it's also the thoughts and intentions of your heart (Heb. 4:12).

Sigh . . .

Nobody gets out of this understanding unscathed.

## The Great Big Lie of Little Bitty Sins

As Christians, we're pretty squishy these days on the gravity of sin. I know this because I'm a Christian and I find myself being cavalier about the blackness of my acts. I focus on the acts and not against whom the act offends. *Oh, this one bout of gluttony's not so bad . . . Even if it goes on for a few weeks, I can get back on track and lose the weight.*

Um . . . No?

I might as well be saying in my heart, *Oh, giving God the middle finger isn't so bad . . . Even if it goes on for a few weeks, I can get back on track and ask His forgiveness because, after all, Jesus died for my sins so that's how we deal with that, right?* May it never be! (Rom. 6:1–7).

Sorry to be crass, but yeah, it's really just that bad.

That's why everyone in the Bible pleads with their listeners and readers to repent. The writers aren't being uptight killjoys, they see sin for the absolute disease of the heart that it is, and they plead for anyone who'll heed their words to turn away from it.

Regardless of how much you believe you're the star of your story, in the end, God is the reason this whole movie exists; it's all for His pleasure (Ps. 24:1). He made the world a pretty place with things to see, smell, touch and taste. He set us in it as part of His masterpiece, not so we could see, smell, touch and taste it alone, but so we could say "Wow, God! You're simply amazing! You made all this stuff out of your head!"

Yet everything He created in all the universes is just a hazy reference to the beauty of His eternal Kingdom: a Kingdom that is a perfect reflection of who He is. That's why letting ourselves be captivated with all we see and experience in this world so that we wander from the path that leads to God is, ultimately, foolishness. This world is not going to last as it is.

Now that you understand the gravity and consequences for sin, I hope you can trust God, who wants to perform the lifesaving operation that will fix your heart. He has just as much at stake with your change as you do. When a person dies, they lose life for all eternity, but when God sees a person die, He loses someone for whom He had compassion (Jonah 4:10-11).

## The Loving Splinter Surgeon

If we think back on our lives we can remember the first splinter removal we endured as a child. The tiny sliver was painful, but the digging around to remove it seemed to be worse. In my case, the only reason I allowed it to continue was because I knew my mother, who was trying her best to remove it, loved me very much. When God seeks to deal with the sins in our heart, He too does it in love, even if the removal of that sin is painful.

While non-Christians may only just be beginning to understand the depth of the disease of sin in their hearts by the consequences they are destined to face, we Christians who grasp this nevertheless persist in doing the very thing God literally hates because the thought of facing the trials in our lives without the comfortable buffer that sin provides is too much to bear.

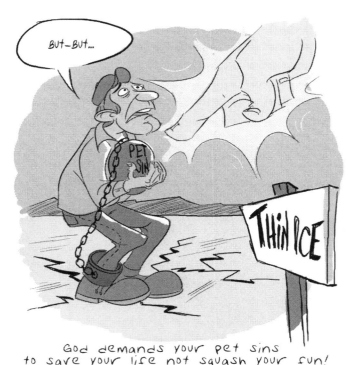

God demands your pet sins to save your life not squash your fun!

God won't let us hold onto our beloved sins forever. They're like the splinter which, if left in place, will cause an infection. He may gently coax you to relinquish your hold on your beloved sin, but if you're stubborn. He may eventually rap your knuckles with His holy yardstick of conviction or consequence.

In the end, when God points out your sin and calls you to repent, it isn't only about you bearing His likeness; He also wants you to learn about His tender love. By His involvement in your life, even in the gnarly bits, He shows His fatherly devotion to you.

There was a time many years ago when I was struggling with understanding God's compassion to me in the midst of working on a very challenging project while also caring for my mother who had cancer. One day, I took her to the hospital for major surgery and then went to straight to work rather than staying to wait with her. My boss, a mercurial man who in the past had been very harsh with me, saw me at my desk and said, "I thought your mother was scheduled for surgery today?"

"She is . . . " I replied in a small, weak voice, "but I was afraid what would happen if I didn't get my work done."

My boss paused in awkward silence then added, "One time my cousin's little girl got really sick . . . She almost died . . . "

After which he stiltedly lurched into my cubicle and surprised me with a stiff hug before he retreated and vanished down the hall. Instantly the words of the summation of the story Jesus told in Luke 18:1–8 sprang to mind. In the story of a poor widow who wins protection, due to her persistence, from a powerful but initially unwilling judge, Jesus concludes " . . . *now, will not God bring about justice for His elect who cry to Him day and night, and will He delay long over them? I tell you that He will bring about justice for them quickly.*" Here I'd found compassion from my boss who was typically harsh toward me and in seeing this, I realized God was so much more compassionate to me, though I doubted His goodness in my pain and fear of the unknown.

If we can trust Him as He carefully helps us remove the sinful infections in our hearts, we can trust God to represent us in the trials that face our lives. We need to turn to Him rather than further feeding our sinful inclinations under the table.

Often, we're so uncomfortable with the unknowns in our life we turn to the comfort of sin instead of running to God who knows all and will provide a shelter in our storms. Why do we think that people or things may have time for us, but God can't be bothered to deal with us in our pain?

If by chance we *do choose* not to sin because it's the right thing to do, we may mistakenly slap a label on any sin struggle and say, "You're bad. The Bible's good. Go do the Bible, you knucklehead, and stop that sinning. You sinner, you—and while you're at it, quit that simpering in pain." That would deny the fact God cares we're human, with hurts and broken dreams. We aren't always seeking pleasure because we're wanton pleasure-worshippers. Sometimes we do it because we're just really, really hurting. We're lonely or disappointed, angry or lost. We want to not hurt, is all. So sin becomes an anesthetic.

The fact is, sinning actually does feel good for a bit, but God knows what we forget when we choose to surrender to sin: The choice to sin doesn't take away the problems; it just pushes them off to a later time. The result is we have to keep sinning to keep from feeling the emotions created by the existence of the trial instead of actually dealing with it where we can (or, where we can't, resting in God's sovereignty, believing that He has orchestrated this event to chip away something harmful to our character).

God wants so much more for us than sin's failed promises to satisfy. He also wants to change the priorities in our hearts so we don't need to run to anything else to make us feel better. However, that often takes time and a lot of hard work. In the midst of our struggle to repent of our sins that have been dredged up by our life circumstances, we need to understand that God tenderly understands our longings. One need only look to the Bible to see the compassion of God expressed through His son Jesus as He acted, *"moved with compassion"* (Matt. 9:36–37; 14:13–14; 15:29–32; 20:29–34; Mark 1:40–41; 6:33–34; Luke 7:11–16). Furthermore, remember that not only is the Holy Spirit's purpose to convict all of sin, He also provides God's children with help (John 14:6; 16:8).

When we mistakenly think God is some stodgy grumpypants who merely demands slavish "thou shalt not" obedience while He stomps with jackboots on our wounded hearts, we miss the fact that in addition to being holy, the Trinity—Father, Son and Spirit—is also love (1 John 4:8). The holy triumvirate isn't sitting in heaven laughing at your pain like some gang of high school bullies in the quad. They know this world is broken because of sin's unchecked rampage, and the Father, Son and Spirit are able to provide comfort because, though everything around us may seem out of control, they know the precise time when this wretched world will be made new. Trust the Holy Trinity the way a small child trusts his father in a crushing crowd. Because the child's papa can see that up ahead is an opening, the child holds onto his hand, knowing that something better than stinky bottoms and swinging fists lies ahead. Just as the child looks up and catches the eye of His daddy and receives a reassuring smile, rest assured, the God who calls you to walk the one path that leads to Him, will provide comfort to you as you do it (2 Cor. 1:3–5). Though it may take time to come into that place of comfort, we need to be patient and obedient as we wait for God's provision.

God is better to us than we are. If it were up to us, we'd settle for the temporary comfort sin provides, rather than patiently persevering through the trials associated with obeying His biblical directives. However, God's best for us is the lasting satisfaction revealed after we've chosen to submit to His transformation in our lives.

I understand if you're reading this book, you're probably suffering from some tremendous pain: a disappointing love life, a bad job, failed health or unfulfilled dreams. Maybe all of them. All you understand is the dull or roaring ache of today as it stretches into the next week and the week after that, down months pouring into years. It's so very overwhelming. Of course you want some relief. You want to put off this surgery until a more convenient time, although this disease is eventually going to kill you.

God knows. And He calls to you in your pain:

> *Come to Me, all who are weary and heavy-laden, and I will give you rest.*
> *Take My yoke upon you and learn from Me, for I am gentle and humble in heart,*
> *and you will find rest for your souls. For My yoke is easy and My burden is light.*
>
> *Matt. 11:28–30*

The life of righteousness is a life that works, and when I say "works," I refer to hard manual labor. That's what yoked animals do: grinding work. Yet Jesus shows in His call to come to Him that He isn't an overbearing taskmaster, but a gentle and humble one who'll give us eventual rest for our souls.

He sees that you're weary and weighed down. He's not standing in His royal throne room saying, "I know your husband just left you after you found out you had breast cancer, and your son is doing drugs with his no-account friends, but suck it up; act right." God who knows the ending of your story knows that the way to a better you is often through the land of obeying while living *in* that pain.

## The Best God for the Job

The God who wants you to let Him perform the heart surgery you need can be trusted to use the tools of circumstances and His instruction in the Bible.

I've long since come to the conclusion the world would be in a horrible place if I were God. I'm not talking about my lack of organization or the fact that I don't have limitless energy, or even my inability to see without glasses (and even with them, not very well). The reason I would make a truly horrible excuse for a god is because people annoy me.

Well, let me rephrase that . . . People's PROBLEMS annoy me. Not all people, though. I can find a weird sense of compassion for those who're younger than me. I see them struggle with their problems, listen to them cry and think, *Poor dear . . . Years from now this won't be so bad. You'll be thankful you missed out on that boy who broke your heart when he took your best friend to the prom because he actually turned out to be a bum, or that you were crushed when the first job you really wanted didn't hire you because it opened up a door for something else, or that your newlywed husband is having a hard go of it right now at his job and you have no idea how to comfort him other than think of ways to make his home a haven. I know beyond a shadow of a doubt that God has a purpose in this and He will grow you through it . . . And, by the way, did you get that meme I sent you?*

However things for which I have no answers disturb me when I encounter them in people around my age. My response is commonly: *Stop it. Stop feeling that way. I know you're hurting, but please, this is messy and I don't know what to do with messy. I've never experienced this brand of mess before and if I have, it's only been once or twice, so I can't say for certain that the only reason I got through that "messy" wasn't because of dumb blind luck . . .*

*Okay. Okay, fine. You're still here. Try this formula . . . Now? No? Why are we here? You just want to whine—er, I mean, talk? Ugh. I dunno. Please run along. Go find someone else to whom God has given the gift of wisdom to handle your messy, cumbersome, potentially not quickly solvable problem.*

Thank heavens we have a God who's not like me or even you.

Our compassion is based on how we lived through our past experiences but God's compassion is based on the future and rests on His ability to accomplish His plans to bring that future to fruition (1 Thess. 5:23–24).

What does this have to do with the insistence that we have a God who sees our sin as so detrimental to us that He vehemently goes for its roots in our hearts? Everything. If we see God with the same short-tempered, inconsiderate flaws we have, we won't ever follow Him. If we're impatient with others, we probably believe God is the same with us. If we refuse to listen with compassion, we can't help but think that God will be just as hard-hearted.

However, God isn't like us. He never walks away from us in frustration when we fail (Heb. 7:22–25). He never loses attention or gets icked-out by our struggles. He hears every little prayer no matter how mundane we think it may be . . . Seriously, *to a God who is infinite, isn't everything mundane?*

God is the best one for the job because of His perfection of character in every facet. His way is an excellent way, even though it may lead through a thorny path at times.

Though we are made in His image, God is so unlike the beings He created because He is perfect. Not only are His ways and thoughts different from our own, so also is the graciousness of His heart toward a repentant sinner (Isa. 55:7–9). Jesus, who is God incarnate, called Peter a rock though he knew the impetuous disciple would soon deny Him three times (Matt. 16:17–18a; 26:69–75; John 21:12–18). Yet He saw the eventual greener pastures He had planned for Peter when he returned. This same God sees us in all our good and bad times. He sees us, and is committed to see us through them.

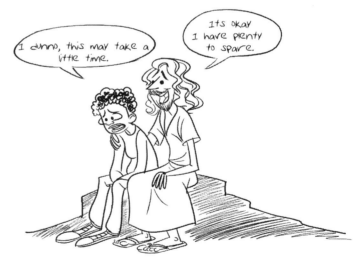

God is infinite. He has all the time in the world to transform you.

God isn't unaware of the rocks of sinful inclination in the field of our lives but those stones and boulders don't frustrate Him, for He who resurrected Jesus from the dead has the power to remove all obstacles to the beauty He longs to create in us. God, being infinite in all things, has great inexhaustible wells of patience. He has perfect love and mercy so that He can walk with us on the course of transformation. He will make sure we get home. He is our loving Father; He committed Himself to care for us when we crawled—dirty, shivering, fearful and weeping—into His lap and asked to be saved.

# He Loved You Before You Were Born

Over the years, I've often heard people say "I have no patience for kids except my own." God isn't like that. Understand that God doesn't just turn on His patience when a person gets saved. He's already patient because that is part of His character (Rom. 9:22–23; 2 Pet. 3:9–13). If He has that kind of patience for those who have nothing but contempt for Him (in the worst cases), as well as for those who just ignore Him (in the least of cases), imagine how much *more* patience He has for those who are truly His children? God has wells of patience for us as Christians, because before we were ever born He chose us (Eph. 1:3-5). If He was longsuffering with us when we were His enemies, He is going to be patient with as we struggle to grow to look like Him as His children.

God says there is only one narrow way to Him, yet understanding that He's gently leading us along that path equips us to move forward and listen to the things I plan to discuss in the next chapter.

Over the years as I've struggled to overcome this issue of my weight, I've encountered people who rigorously asserted that the sins that promote obesity are not as bad as other sins. They wag their fingers at promiscuity and blasphemy, but think what I'm about to discuss in the next chapter isn't such a big bad deal. They mistakenly classify their sins on the sin-o-meter as light (if they call it a sin at all) and others' sins as heavy. As I have been saying, isn't all ungodliness the same to a God who's holy? I am too simple to understand the finer points of a holy God's execution of righteous judgment for various sins, but I do know that *all sin will send you to hell* and Jesus' death is sufficient to pay for all sin, *regardless of what it is.*

So imagine the broken body of Christ lying amidst the rubble of stolen goods, used condoms, aborted babies, discarded weapons AND extra plates from multiple helpings, then you will begin to see the shame of the sin you call "not as bad as others." If Jesus died for everything, then His death truly is love. Then you can also imagine Him standing up from that pile of refuse, coming to you with His arms wide open and saying, "Here, take my robe of righteousness. I'm giving it to you . . . "

When we come to see how totally depraved we are for the pet sin we feed under the table, we will to begin to grasp the breadth of Jesus' sacrifice. Christ was tempted in all things and didn't fail. It wasn't that He was tempted in all things and only succeeded in withstanding the big things. It's not like Jesus died a little. He died the whole way. Dead. We miss the wells of grace God has lavished on us when we lessen the severity of the reason for the death of Christ by classifying some as "little sins" or even rationalizing them away in the first place.

To paraphrase Matthew 8:36 it is possible to lose a hundred pounds and still lose your soul. That's why I called this chapter "The Death Row Dieter." God is concerned about your heart that put you in the place of judgment. When you address the sin in your heart, it clears the way for you to move forward in obedience. Are you ready to address the sins of your heart that may be contributing to your long-term size? If so, you're ready to go to the next chapter and take the lampshade off the elephant in the room.

• • • • • • •

*Ev'ry day the Lord Himself is near me*
*With a special mercy for each hour;*
*All my cares He fain would bear, and cheer me,*
*He whose name is Counselor and Pow'r.*
*The protection of His child and treasure*
*Is a charge that on Himself He laid:*
*"As thy days, thy strength shall be in measure,"*
*This the pledge to me He made.*

*Help me then in eve'ry tribulation*
*So to trust Thy promises, O Lord,*
*That I lose not faith's sweet consolation*
*Offered me within Thy holy Word.*
*Help me, Lord, when toil and trouble meeting,*
*E'er to take, as from a father's hand,*
*One by one, the days, the moments fleeting,*
*Till I reach the promised land."* [7]

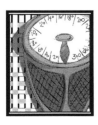

# Take A-Weigh

- God wants to change you from the inside.
- Sin is gravely deadly.
- God's way is the only way to eternal life and overcoming sin.
- God is compassionate in helping us to change.

[7] From "Day by Day," A.L. Skoog and Carolina Sandell, lyrics 1865, public domain.

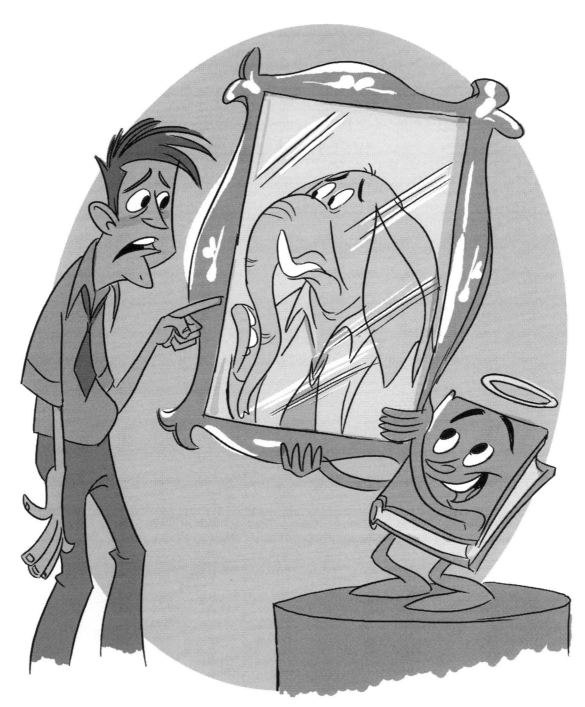

Mirror, mirror of God's word.
Let me accept what I just heard.

Chapter 5

# Greed: The Elephant in the Room

> *For many walk, of whom I often told you, and now tell you even weeping, that they are enemies of the cross of Christ, whose end is destruction, whose god is their appetite, and whose glory is in their shame, who set their minds on earthly things. For our citizenship is in heaven, from which also we eagerly wait for a Savior, the Lord Jesus Christ; who will transform the body of our humble state into conformity with the body of His glory, by the exertion of the power that He has even to subject all things to Himself.* Phil. 3:18–21

An older woman once told me, "People eat with their eyes before they eat with their mouths." With that, I began my quest to make both delicious and visually appealing dishes. The problem is I'm tremendously clumsy. No matter how determined I am to present things well, I end up with disappointing results. Well at least it tastes good, right?

Once I was tasked with baking a birthday cake. It was going to be raison d'etre! I wasn't going to fail. After preparing the perfect recipe and decorating it reasonably well, all that remained was transporting it.

Why I did it on a cake stand is beyond me.

I think I made it a block before it happened. Centrifugal force. My hands glued to the wheel, I watched in horror as I turned left and the beautiful cake rocked forward on its glass stand and ever so slowly . . . Fell. Off. The. Seat.

It had strawberries on it and everything. What was once a thing of beauty was now a broken, floury lump mixed with whipped cream, twigs, leaves and dirt from the car mat.

We have discussed that sin is missing the mark or wandering from the law of God. God isn't a party pooper. He knows how things function best because He created every-thing. Remember, "The Bible isn't a book of don'ts. It's a book of do's." God gives us good gifts, but we turn them into sin when we take any good thing and use it out of the context for which it was intended.

While you might eat a beautiful cake on a china plate, you'd never spoon it from a car mat mixed with the twigs and shoe grime no matter how good it tastes. Yet you would consider premarital sex, taking someone's life unjustly, or gleefully participating in the sin that contributes to your long-term weight gain because it feels good.

## Appearance Versus Appetite

Being fat isn't the sin. *It's the consequence of sinning.* Just like having a baby out of wedlock isn't sin, but sleeping with someone before you're married to him or her is.

In the time since I started this book there have been various articles regarding the sin I'm about to discuss in this chapter, which encourages me greatly. *(Okay . . . I'm not making an issue out of a non-issue.)* While a lot of times the writer has been praised for "finally talking about a taboo subject," I'm saddened at how many people viciously retaliate, insisting everything from, "This isn't a sin!" to "You can't say this is as bad as perverted sexual immorality!" or "how dare you fat-shame us!"

Big sad face . . .

I can only offer my life—or more specifically how GOD worked through my life—as an example. I weigh in on this subject humbly because I remember my years of fighting the conviction of my sin. However there's hope when you finally understand sin is sin, whether it's a "small" or "large" one and that being called to repent of it isn't fat-shaming you because thin people can also participate in this sin.

Appearance means more to humans than it does to God. Jesus didn't walk among the people He created looking like either a runway model or a Muscle Beach meathead. Instead He dwelled on this earth in a completely unremarkable form. People weren't meant to be drawn to His packaging, but to His preaching (Isa. 53:2; Matt. 4:15–17). Therefore the purpose of these pages isn't so you'll be a hottie in a new body—but so the effects of your sin (how you appear physically) won't obfuscate the message of Christ's redemption of the lost.[8] When you submit to God from your heart and gradually change so that all the people in your life see His rule in your life, they take note of how God takes the unlovely, the castoffs, the weak and the foolish, and makes something from their broken lives (1 Cor. 1:26–31). Your repentance makes you a living gospel tract to your friends and family who don't believe God exists or, if He does, that He doesn't really care.

We are to aim to have a heart submitted to the Lord in all things, even the food we put into our mouths. Take a look at the Lord's Prayer and see that He exhorted His followers to

---

[8] 1 Samuel 16:7 acknowledges that people judge visually. Sometimes they can be cruel. God sees everyone He's saved as they will be in heaven and loves us because of the work He's doing in us. We shouldn't be discouraged that people judge us when we're overweight. Instead we should be excited that we get the opportunity to show them, "Boom, Baby—God IS real! Just look what He's done in my heart, because it changed my life!"

submit even their requests for food to their Father in heaven (Matt. 6:11). We need food to live; it's not just a luxury. A quick Internet search on how long a person can last without food comes up with twenty-one days. Jesus did forty, but going beyond that means death. So if we're to bring the very thing we need to survive before God, we're asking Him to keep us alive. Yet it's very easy to turn this thing He provides for our survival into a trip to the fair.

That's where one begins to sin—and remember, this sin is no less deadly than any other.

While we'll discuss increasing physical activity and eating choices in chapters 11 through 13, just exercising or dieting away the long-term physical effects of this sin isn't actually dealing with the heart sin itself; that's just dealing with the consequence. To deal with *sanctifying your appetite* God wants us to understand these things:

1) God is our master—not our appetites.

2) God made food to be thankfully enjoyed, but not overindulgently.

3) God's mercies are new every morning; He's forgiving when we sin.

Before we go on to the specific "elephant" we've been ignoring, I want to lay a little groundwork to help you understand the physical mechanics behind weight.

# The Physiology of Fatness

Recently I was hiking with some friends. One of them asked me why it was so easy for me (and others like me) to lose and gain weight so quickly. . . mostly the gain part. The reason, I explained, is because of the wheres and hows of fat storage. There's a lot of fascinating research filled with scientific words which explains what makes people fat and how they stay there. Some of it involves carbon dating and cold war nuclear testing, believe it or not. But the simplest way of thinking about it is this: Living creatures have little cell suitcases filled with fat to keep them alive. Everyone's born with them. Where the fat suitcases are on a person's body is determined by gender. Fat tends to be stored in certain areas of the body, and it contributes to what makes men look like men and women look like women. However the problem comes when, like everything in life, there's too much of a good thing. We need to store *some* fat because we're not eating *all* the time. So between meals, the body lives off what's been stored from the previous meal, basically like the gas in the tank of a car. The problem comes not merely from the way people keep cramming fat in those cellular suitcases, but in how many cellular suitcases they have. You see, *everyone* has fat suitcases in their body, but fat people have *more* of them. (And some research says that their suitcases may indeed be steamer trunks.) Folks tend to build all the storage they'll ever have by their teen years. They can never lose them once they've built them, they can only shrink their contents. Interestingly, the body replaces about eight to ten percent of their fat suitcases yearly so the stores are at a constant balance. Hooray for the efficiency of this machine in which we live!

In a perfect world, we have the storage we need to keep ourselves alive and nothing, no nothing, interferes with our ability to keep going through the course of the day because we can unpack what we need from our carry-on luggage. A problem arises, however, when we have more things stuffed into our suitcases than we need.

For the most part, once people reach adulthood, they very rarely become obese. That's why childhood obesity is such a huge deal. When children get fat, they're actually building extra suitcases that'll last a lifetime. A friend asked me if I could've lost the extra fat storage if I'd had liposuction, and I discovered that while it's possible, it amounts to a drastic measure to take care of the problem that doesn't solve the underlying reason why you cram too much stuff in your suitcase in the first place. While it takes a lot of work, a person *can* actually add fat suitcases after they get older if they are excessive eaters (and in the case of people who get lipo, though the weight may not return in force to the treated areas, it will make the untreated areas larger).

Excess fat in your body decreases the hormone that makes you feel satiated, which is why it takes obese people longer to feel full. Basically, the job of the hormone called leptin is to tell your body, "Okay, you've had enough to sustain you beyond the act of getting food into your system— now go out and be productive!" For some reason, being fatter suppresses the manufacture of this hormone. That's not the only bit of irony—*dieting* actually increases the hormone ghrelin, which makes a person hungry! Simply stated, whether you eat too much or too little, your body will want more. Which is why merely going on yet another diet isn't necessarily going to provide you lasting satisfaction. Okay, that's the science stuff simplified for people like me who don't like science. You're welcome.

The one notion I was repeatedly confronted with in my limited research was the conclusion of "science," namely that people are helpless to overcome their biology; they're doomed to an endless cycle of limited success and great failures in their battle against their weight. One article went on to posit the idea that attitudes need to change toward the obese to favor the notion that obesity isn't due to lack of self-control or willpower, but because of biological factors people have been saddled with in their childhoods.

All that knowledge and research, only to come to the conclusion, "Pfft. Too bad, them's just the breaks. Maybe one day we'll come up with a solution, but don't hold your breath because even then, the body's pretty tricky and will find a way around the fix." The world has all that learning, and yet no real answers (2 Tim. 3:1–7). As with so many other issues in today's culture, we're told that obesity isn't a choice, but rather a dictate of our biology— we're born that way. Or if not that, at least it's not our fault, but the fault of our parents or our environment. How hopeless...

Yet if we go to the sinful source of what packs on the pounds, the Bible has the answer to the question "wretched man that I am! Who will deliver me from this body of death?" found in the apostle Paul's statement of praise: *"Thanks be to God through Jesus Christ our Lord!"* (Rom. 7:25),

Do I have your attention? Does God?

I hope so, because His word lovingly reveals His commands that instruct us how to be like Him in the area of our appetite, and an appetite submitted to Him produces results in due time (James 4:7-10).

## Born This Way—But Not the Way That You Think

I opened this chapter with the physiology behind fat, but now I'd like to go a little deeper to what drives some of us to eat more than we need. This affects both those who show the results of sin by long-term weight gain and those who don't.

While I'm not waving a flag, falling lockstep into the "born this way" crowd, I believe we all have besetting sins which plague us. That's why some teetotalers commit adultery, while other faithful spouses are alcoholics. My mother told me that when I was just a toddler, I was still adorable and normal-sized, she saw I had a voracious appetite. She told me once she fed me a dozen to a dozen-and-a-half eggs one at a time to see how many I would eat before I stopped. Later as a four-year-old, I wouldn't eat my favorite blueberry turnover because my stomach hurt. I would've gone on like that all day, but my Aunt Frank insisted I eat something to make myself feel better . . . and it was then I discovered I'd been hungry all along. So having a voracious appetite and an inability to determine what was hunger created a perfect storm to pack on the pounds as I grew. Maybe you too have some issue which has broken your eat switch or you have always had the inclination to overindulge, but just because you or I are drawn to particular besetting sins or have various handicaps doesn't mean we must be slaves to obey them (Rom. 6:12–20).

God has given us the power in Christ to identify and turn from our besetting sins. However before we can turn from them we have to ask and answer for ourselves the hard question . . .

If it's not health-related, what makes people obese or even a little overweight? Furthermore, what prevents them from losing the weight, or if they succeed in losing it, what prevents them from keeping it off? What is this sin that affects both those who show it as well as even the people who don't show its effects? The Bible says its greed.

In my testimony I mentioned Ephesians 5:3–5 because it lists traits that characterized my life before I was saved and in some cases after, *the chief one for me being greed*. While I will move on to the further reasons for long-term weight gain, I'm starting with this facet of sin so that those of you who might want to find an excuse, can't. It's not only poor eating habits that keep us big; it's our desire to eat more than we need.

We often think of greed to describe the miser who amasses fortunes while others are needy or collectors who take great delight in filling their rooms with goods no matter how many things they have, to the point that they have to build more rooms or rent storage. We look at those people with a certain quiet outrage:

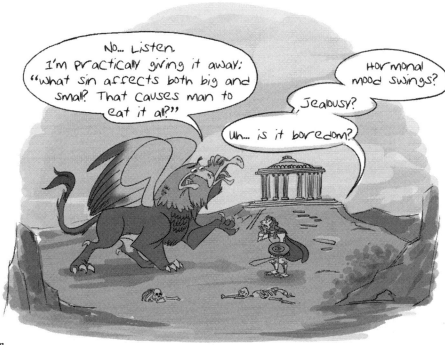

The thirteenth unknown labor of Hercules.

*If only they took what was enough for them and no more. If only they thought more of others and less of themselves . . .* Meanwhile we ladle a second helping of Wes's secret recipe cream corn on our already wilted paper plates. It's more than the inordinate love of mammon and materials that constitutes greed. If greed is in a person's heart, it'll find its way to be expressed whether it's in wanting more money or things than we can ever use in a lifetime, or looking with envious eyes at the amazing spouse someone else has, or having extra helpings at the church potluck. As fat Christians, we look at some expressions of greed as repugnant while ours gets a pass, but God says, *"You shall not have any other gods before me"* (Ex. 20:3) because He sees all workings of greed the same. He sees them as idolatry.

The biblical definition of the word "greed" found in Colossians 3:5 and Ephesians 5:5 means a greedy desire to have more, to have avarice or to be covetous. Which being interpreted, means we want more than what we have; more than what's given to us; or, if someone else has it and we don't, we want that, too. We're too impatient to have it later; we want it all now. We're like little babies who say "Me, me, me," or like the leech's daughters who cry, " 'Give,' 'Give' " (Prov. 30:15). So that's why that second piece of pie after we're no longer hungry constitutes the sin of greed, and according to the word of God is on par with immorality, impurity, passion, and evil desire. (In Ephesians 5:5, the New International Version exchanges the word for coveting found in the NASB with the word "greed." Either way, the sin has its roots in the same source.)

God's law is black and white and the not shades of grey like we like to paint it. We who are believers have the assurance that our sins are forgiven, but that doesn't mean we can go on walking in the areas over which God has put a giant red circle slash. Once we're saved, we're called to see the black and white of God for what it is. See it, and flee from it—and not be like the Norman Rockwell Saturday Evening Post painting of the woman who's trying to tip the scale up while the butcher tries to hold it down. For a Christian, the gospel that produces salvation means nothing to us if it doesn't also lead us to obedient change.

So for those of us who don't battle with acquiring too much stuff but with eating too much, let's see what the Bible says about the sin of greed as it expresses itself through gluttony.

## Big-Eyed Greedy-Gut

When I was a little girl, my great uncle occasionally chanted, "Big-eyed greedy-gut. Eat the whole world up . . . " I didn't understand it at the time, but he was playfully alluding to my excessive eating. He was an affable man who always played practical jokes on us, and so I just saw the rhyme as part of his shtick. But God doesn't joke when it comes to sin. Though He will discipline us for disobeying his commands, He's a loving Father who tells us what He wants from us so we can know His mind. With that in mind, we need to come to an understanding that God isn't down with gluttony.

What is gluttony?

Merriam-Webster's online dictionary defines gluttony as "the act or habit of eating or drinking too much." [9]

We in Western culture have expanded the meaning of the word based on our attitudes toward morbidly obese people. Western culture sees a glutton as someone who's ugly, lazy and probably isn't very smart. Based on this expanded definition, some people decide an obese person is someone who isn't worth their time. Meanwhile those same people who disdainfully look down on the overweight apply a lighter definition of gluttony to themselves to mean someone who occasionally overindulges at the holidays or on special occasions. They reason, A *few extra days in my yoga pants isn't the same as your taking up two seats on the airplane, so out of the emergency aisle, you dumb fatso!*

. . . Wow . . .

The shifting opinions and standards of man.

So we don't go to man to define what essentially is a holy rebellion against God. Let's go to God Himself. According to the Old Testament, a glutton is one who makes light of, squanders or is lavish with something, while the New Testament defines the word glutton as

---

[9] From Merriam-Webster's Collegiate® Dictionary, 11th Edition ©2015, Merriam-Webster, Inc. (www.Merriam-Webster.com).

a gormandizer or "someone who is all stomach."

Nice . . .

Well . . . not really . . .

However it sure does picture what's going on in my head when I keep eating past full. As if I'm trying to make my whole body be storage for what I'm eating. *Who needs lungs? Or a heart? Make room for more pizza!*

So you see the reason why gluttony is more than just a fat person's problem. Everyone is capable of it; some people can just get away with it because their metabolism is faster.

The Bible says with boldness: These people who do this gluttony, these are the results from their acts as a glutton. As if to say you are what you are because *you're an overeater,* not you are what you are because you just overate.

Participating in gluttony does have its consequences. Doing a quick search of the Bible comes up with some pretty bleak pronouncements for gluttons—and none of them are based on looks.

Proverbs warns people to not keep company with gluttons or drunkards and says those who practice such things will eventually find themselves in drowsiness and poverty (Prov. 23:20–21). Later it says keeping company with gluttons is a humiliation to one's parents (Prov. 28:7). For the *pièce de résistance,* Titus 1:10–12 lumps gluttons into the category of *"rebellious men, empty talkers and deceivers . . . always liars, evil beasts, lazy . . . "*

Ahhh . . . good times.

So we see the Bible doesn't look kindly on the whole "super-size" mentality we've grown to accept as normal. Yet I've never heard the subject discussed from the pulpit. Sunday after Sunday, pastors will stand behind their lecterns and admonish adultery, look down on lust, lower the boom on lying—but excuse everyone after the sermon's amen to the church potluck to enjoy a piece of pie . . . and cookies, and three pieces of Sister-So-and-So's award-winning fried chicken.

God will not be mocked. Whatever a man sows, he reaps (Gal. 6:7).

God wants all of us: why do we think that the One who commands us to take our thoughts, which are as ethereal as smoke, captive is going to turn a blind eye to our excessive appetites that are as tangible as a stone in our shoe. God calls us to submit even what we eat to Him (1 Cor. 10:31).

While gluttony finds the flower of its expression in eating too much, its roots go much deeper, for it grows from seed of coveting.

The Bible defines "coveting" as *having an excessive desire or longing.*

Having desires is not a bad thing. The Bible assures us if we delight in the Lord He'll give us the desires of our heart (Ps. 37:4) and that God opens His hand and satisfies the desires of every living thing (Ps. 145:16).

However desire becomes excessive when we want what we want for its own sake and ignore the One who's given it. It's a matter of the heart to which we can easily succumb to unless we're on guard. So many times, I've started being thankful to God for sushi, but ended veering off on the path of gratitude into the trap of my lust for how awesome a second serving of monkfish liver would be . . . (Okay, maybe not a conventional covet.

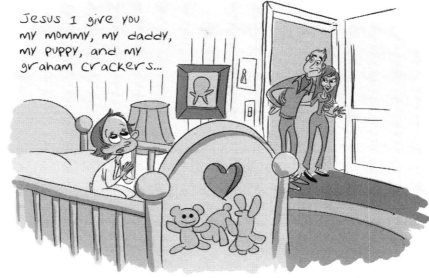

Insert your prepacked-cream-filled-snack-cakes, crispy-salty-puffy chips, or your mom's pot roast here.) In this way, we can make an idol out of the desires God fulfills.

Coveting/greed/gluttony becomes an issue of worshipping something other than God. In doing this we worship the creation, not the Creator, and God justifiably gives us over to the consequences of our choice (Rom. 1:25). It's not just the worldly ones in their worship of sex who suffer the consequences of disease and loneliness, the ones we in the church are so quick to dismiss with self-righteousness. No, God also "gives over" to their consequences those who worship at the altar of second helpings.

This issue of idolatry toward food doesn't only cover eating too much, it covers eating for the wrong reasons. When we turn to food to deal with emotions or circumstances we face, this constitutes greed as well. I know there are times I've eaten when I wasn't hungry, trying to fill some emptiness due to discontentment, boredom or sorrow instead of turning to God for comfort and accepting His plans for my life. This too is sin. The same God who fulfills our desires says he does it *in due season*. Therefore it's presumptuous of us to be discontented with the season we're in. We need to prayerfully bring our longings to Him and, as I said earlier, change the things we can. We need to accept that God has a plan in the things we cannot change, one that will be revealed in His perfect time. Is this easy? Nope. But faith is like a muscle, it won't grow unless it's worked. The more we prayerfully turn to God to ask for help to accept His will instead of turning to food, the less challenging our struggle to wait for Him will become.

In engaging in these sins, the danger isn't only the consequences of disease and alienation from others as it affects our bodies: the bigger impact is how coveting affects our relationship with God.

Don't get me wrong. Once you're saved, you're saved. However besetting sins like long-term greed, when allowed to linger in your life, are like taking polyfill batting, wrapping it around your head and then putting a bucket on top of it for good measure. All the while you wonder, *Why can't I hear God?*

While I say your unwillingness to submit your appetite to God does not determine whether or not you're saved, I'd humbly encourage you to ask yourself the hard question: if you're not even willing to try to repent in this area, do you indeed have the power within you to change as given to all who believe in the gospel? After all, God resurrected Jesus from the dead, for goodness sakes, He certainly has the ability to give you the desire to put down your fork when you're satisfied. That is unless you're still dead in your trespasses and sins and your appetite is like a fire, which can never have enough (Prov. 30:15b–16).

If we find a lack of contentment in the amount we have on our plates before us, or if we're double-minded and can't make a decision as to which thing we'll eat so we just take both—or if we eat in emotional response and not because we're hungry; we're being greedy, covetous, gluttons.

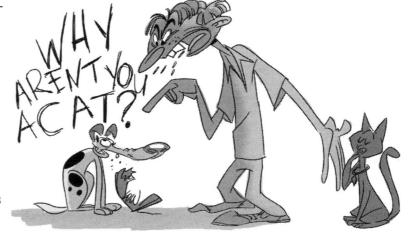

In the previous chapter, I wrote how no sin is greater or smaller than another, but how can I make that assertion when eating two pizzas seems so much less harmful than murdering a room full of school children?

I can say this because all sins share the same root: pride. I don't mean the kind of pride that says, "I'm better-looking than the average Joan"; I mean the sort that claims "I know what's best for me and no one can tell me otherwise—especially God." The Bible asserts when people rely on their own way, it's going to end poorly for them. And when I say "poorly" I mean deadly (Prov. 16:25). For the first thing new Christians do is to renounce their thinking that they know what's best . . . well, in theory they do. It may take longer in some areas than in others, but the long-term goal for God's children is to stop thinking our practices are right and to trust Him that His ways will lead us away from death.

Believe me I KNOW how hard this is. I struggle with it constantly. I'm thankful for God's grace to forgive, and more than that, I'm thankful for His firm discipline to mold me and teach me how to obey Him better.

# Partial Total Control

When we Christians first approach Him for forgiveness, we come with the realization God wants to control all of us, and we're willing to give all of us to Him. However, as He starts poking around in the treasure chest of our heart, we discover that all of us actually means *all of us,* and we slam the lid shut on that one little thing in the corner of the treasure chest as we think, *Well, that one thing is so little, it won't really matter . . .*

Ehhh . . . well, it does.

God doesn't want halfhearted commitment. He wants the whole show. For you cat lovers (which, sorry, I'm not) He's like that cat who stands outside your door in the still of the night, sticking his paw underneath it.

Fubbidy, fubbidy fubidy fub . . .

*Let me in, let me in,* He insists as He paws at the door of your heart with His giant omnipotent hand.

God always gets His way. If you're truly His own child, He WILL get into your treasure chest no matter how tightly you've closed and tried to hide it with other things, and the genius that He is, *you'll willingly give Him every last bit of its contents.* He's invested far too much in you to let that moldy, mucky thing you're protecting—for that's what your beloved last treasure is—remain. To you it looks like a pile of rubies, but God knows it's actually a pile of dung. Why do we get so confused about this?

The Bible answers the question of "Why do people sin?" with "Because it's pleasurable." So for the purposes of this chapter, I'll ask the question "Why are we greedy/gluttonous?" and show how we prayerfully need to change our attitudes in those areas:

1) Because food tastes good.
2) Because food makes us happy when we're sad.
3) Because food is entertaining when we're bored.
4) Because eating is a situation we can control.
5) Because eating is a reminder of some past pleasant thing.
6) Because eating is all the hope we have.
7) Because we don't know we can sinfully eat.

I wish I could just do away with sinning and move on in life, but God is more interested in what replaces my transgressions than just removing them. I suppose that's why at times I struggle to stay on the path. It's not enough to stop doing those things that give us pleasure in the sin that makes us fat; we need to replace those reasons with God as the answer.[10]

1) We need to taste and see that the Lord is good (Ps. 34:8–10).
2) We need to find that happy is the man who has made the Lord his God (Pss. 40:1–5; 146).
3) We need to realize we're created for specific tasks and pursue them (2 Tim. 2:20–21).
4) We need to recognize that God's in control of all circumstances—both good and bad (Rom. 8:28).
5) We need to express thankfulness for everything God has given us (1 Thess. 5:18).
6) We need to find our hope in the world to come and not in this one (Rom. 8:18–25).
7) We need to learn what pleases the Lord (Eph. 5:15–17).

In the end God wants your repentance in the area of your unchecked appetite, but He doesn't make it complicated. Since greed/gluttony is eating too much, He just asks us to eat what we need and when we need it. The above list is the attitudes we need to prayerfully cultivate as we live. Walking in them takes practice and patience and remembering that God is always gracious and forgiving when we ask His forgiveness when we fail.

## Your Gentle Mahout

The term the "Elephant in the Room" comes from the idea that the only way to deny something as large as an elephant in your room is to ignore that it's there. I titled this chapter, "The Elephant in the Room" because the reason so many of us have become fat and remain so is simply because of our greed. That's the elephant: eating too much. Yes, there are those who have health issues that prevent them from losing weight quickly and I don't want to cause anyone to feel judged. However I hope by now you understand in this book about weight, I'm more interested in losing the life-killing sin of fat in your heart than the fat in your saddle bags (*although I want those gone too*) .

But I want to be gentle. Just because I respond better to a spiritual two-by-four upside

---

[10] The list with verses is by no means exhaustive. These are just the few that I came up off the top of my head to show God has an answer for every question of sin we will face.

my head, doesn't mean everyone is like me. I don't want to place another discouraging heavy load on your spiritual backs. Whether its twenty pounds to lose or a hundred and sixty-two, you may have received so many directions on how to tackle this weighty issue that you feel as if the eyes of all your friends and random strangers who're watching you will be disappointed when you fail . . . a-gain. Now here I come, seeming to add One. Thing. More.

The first time I went on a long training hike, my friend MJ assayed my backpack filled with most of the things I'd need for our eventual ascent to the base of the summit of Mount Whitney. The first thing she removed was the ten pounds of dirt I'd loaded into grocery bags to simulate the food we "might" be carrying. That was the obvious. However the items she removed which weren't as obvious were the redundant objects, or things that were just too heavy because there were actually lighter versions of them she would loan me. She went through each item and carefully but good-naturedly educated me on how to lighten my load. In the end, I had only what I needed.

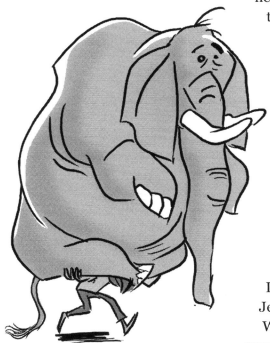

I'm okay... Really.

Allow me to be your MJ; I want to lighten your load, not add to it. I'm pleading with you to throw away everything else: the banishing of foods; the going on fasts; anything you've tried and learned in the past, if it doesn't contribute to trusting this one thing that will work for you. Toss it all out of your spiritual backpack. Seek to submit your appetite to God and repent of your greed and your weight will take care of itself in due time.

Above all in this call to run from this sin, I want to direct you to the gentlest mahout of all: Jesus the Lamb of God.

When I first started obeying God's call to quit being greedy, I remembered the plain and simple truth of Jesus' claim when He said when you've seen me you've seen the Father (John 14:9). Jesus was the expression of God and His love on earth. He was long-suffering, acquainted with sorrows, tempted in all things and yet not falling into temptation. He was compassionate, a healer, a lover of children, a confronter of the self-righteous and a sacrifice for the sins of the world. He was all of these things in love and grace. Now He's seated at the right hand of His Father in heaven, and Jesus still carries all those attributes. Nothing He does is random, chaotic or out of order. He's powerful but restrained. He is perfect but His perfection doesn't crush those who are weak. He knows all and generously gives people information to let them come to their own conclusions. He could be the biggest bully in all of known creation, yet He restrains Himself for a greater plan to redeem mankind.

Let's look at Christ's example of self-control. Self-control is not merely restraining oneself from doing wrong. Self-control is humbling one's self under the control of a loving and powerful God who has a remarkably fabulous plan that's sometimes accomplished through pain. Who likes pain? Show of hands? Not me.

On earth, Jesus was meek and He demonstrated the most supreme act of self-control, because as God, He held all the power in all the worlds to destroy all of mankind as they raged against Him, but as he hung on the cross and died for their sins, instead He whispered, *"Father, forgive them; for they do not know what they are doing"* (Luke 23:34). In this, Jesus demonstrated His inexhaustible love, but not only that; He also showed us the example of self-control that He wants us to follow. For in willingly choosing to die on the cross, Jesus surrendered the control of His self in order that the Father's will might be done (Luke 22:42; Phil. 2:5–8).

Looking at what He did for us, I again plead with you to return to the gospel that expresses the enormous heart God has for you—and that directs you how to live.

When we attempt to control our lives by our own set of standards, we miss the bigger picture of God's plan: to give us endurance in this life and make us more like Jesus (James 1:2-4; Rom. 8:28–29). He knows it's for the best that you're still single at an older age when all your friends are married, or you're in a lousy job you can't escape. He knows that it is advantageous when you're down to your last pennies or your heart is broken over a rebellious child or even that your spouse has died. He knows that ultimately it will be for your good that you are sick or scared or persecuted. Based on Christ's example, which led Him to a painful and shameful death on the cross, we too must trust the Father's bigger plan for our lives beyond the pain we currently endure. We need to trust Him who is our sufficiency and not run to extra helpings to ease our pain.

I understand why it's so tempting to live apart from God's control. Life is so hard, and doing what we want with abandon is something of an anesthetic. However doing what we want, if it's outside God's will, is sin. Ugh—it hurts me to write those words. It seems so harsh—but sometimes hard things need to be said if it's the loving thing to do.

## The Lover of Our Headstrong Hearts

I have a young friend who's got lots of potential but she's slightly headstrong. Therefore, anything that smacks of advice is met with a cheerful but perfunctory, "No, lectures." At one point I asked her for prayer for a situation that was changing in my life and she was alarmed.

As she sought to figure out why my situation was changing, she connected a character flaw she'd observed in my past with the potential source of my current situation and she began to encourage me to change in that area. She was so insistent that I acknowledge and repent of my sin that she missed giving me the directions on the highway, and we had to take the long way home! As I later thought about her response to my problem I couldn't help but smile; she wanted no advice herself but gave me an earful, yet it wasn't because she wanted to cause me harm. Though it made me feel uncomfortable because what she said would mean more work for me, I understood that she had said those things because she cared for me, saw my potential destruction, and wanted to turn me from it.

God, in His command to avoid greed, gluttony and coveting, is like my friend. Even though it hurts to have to apply His commands, He only makes them because He cares for us, sees our potential destruction and wants to turn us from it.

To begin to lose weight, you must accept both God's will for your life in the events as they reveal themselves through the course of the day, as well as God's will for your life as He reveals it to you through the Bible.

God knows how hard it is to accept His will, because Jesus lived the same struggles we face. Go to Him in prayer in your times of wrestling with His will and ask Him for help to accept and live by it. He will joyfully give you aid.

## Sending the Pachyderm Packing

So where do you fall in this spectrum of sin? Do you see the elephant in your room as something you need to show the door, or are you just planning on putting a larger lampshade and some throw pillows on it? The first step to losing weight is more than joining a club or weight loss program: It's as easy as ceasing to add too much fuel to the fire that keeps you fat. If you choose to ignore God's direction for how you should eat, you need to ask yourself, *Do I even care about God?*

When I decided to give God control of my appetite despite the circumstances in my life, I didn't actually feel like doing it. Not that I was antagonistic to it, I just was . . . ambivalent. I knew the right thing to do, but I didn't feel like doing it. As a Christian I took a hard look at my life and realized I was sinning in the area of having a greedy, idolatrous, gluttonous, and covetous appetite. The Bible says, *"Therefore bear fruit in keeping with repentance"* (Matt. 3:8). So repenting meant fighting against eating too much to make myself feel better.

In the end, the reason I was able to start repenting in this area and continue, as well as the reason I'm able to resume when I have a relapse into sin, is my growing relationship with God. Without becoming more and more intimate with Him, it's impossible to sustain wanting to do His will.

Up to this point I've written a lot about what God wants from us and that might be a bit daunting, but it's only daunting if you see Him like Zeus, sitting on his Olympian throne, aloof from his tiny subjects, capriciously hurling down lightning bolts. God isn't like the mythic Greek gods. While we still must wait to see Him as clearly as Adam and Eve once did, He has personally given us an invitation to know Him better (Pss. 34:11-22; John 1:9-13, 6:37; Heb 4:14-16; James 4:7-8). In taking advantage of that access pass to the throne room of grace, we find His commands becoming less burdensome. As we set about deepening our relationship with God, we see the reasons to obey Him—not to win His love, but to continue to discover how much He loves us already.

Jesus said the Father seeks those who long to know him in spirit and in truth (John 4:23). How do you get to that place? We'll talk about that in our next chapter. For now, let's make a decision to get that pachyderm packing, shall we?

**Write down some of your reasons why you've gained weight and why you're still overweight. Look over your list and see the good things God has given you that you've turned into idols. Confess them to God.**

· · · · · · ·

*Dear Lord, I still struggle with this issue. It's not enough to be able to wear smaller clothes and have people notice so that I can give you the praise. It's not enough to lose the weight. People in the world do that every day. I confess that I struggle with reining in my appetite because I love food so much. Help me, Lord, (and help those reading this book) to learn to love you more. Please forgive me. I am so weak and love this world and the things in it so much. Help me to see beyond those foods I love or those circumstances that disappoint me so that I run to food for comfort. Not just so I will run to You for comfort instead, but so I will rest in the circumstance, good or bad, as temporary in light of not only what may be waiting for me around the corner as ordained by You, but also the world to come where I will be with you. Help me to value eternity with You more than the temporary sensation of what delights my taste buds.*

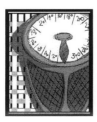

# Take A-Weigh

- Our bodies are perfectly designed for storing/burning food.
- Greed + gluttony + coveting = sin that promotes long-term weight gain.
- We're greedy when we eat too much or for the wrong reasons.
- Jesus demonstrates how we are to turn over our lives to God.
- God's call to quit sinning in your appetite is because He loves you.

# Food for Thought

*"Submit therefore to God. Resist the devil and he will flee from you. Draw near to God and He will draw near to you. Cleanse your hands, you sinners; and purify your hearts, you double-minded. "* James 4:7-8

This chapter is challenging. For those who *have health issues that frustrate your attempt to change your weight* the temptation might arise to dig in your heels. You might insist that your weight isn't a result of sin, but a result of factors beyond your control. You don't want to be judged on the contents of your heart by what people can see with their eyes.

I agree. Let me remind you again. God's admonition to repent in this area affects both the stout and the stick thin. It extends to those who can drop five pounds without a thought and those who have to fight five months for one pound. Remember it's not about the weight; it's about learning to worship God and not food which is His creation.

We must come to the place where we acknowledge our sin before we can repent of it. From there we can run to God for help. Take a few moments to answer these questions so you have an open heart as you proceed to the remaining chapters of this book.

- **On what occasions are you most tempted to overeat?**
- **Where are you as far as acknowledging your overeating as sinful?**
- **How does this chapter change your idea of what is potentially causing your weight issues?**
- **If you have objections to the idea of overeating as being sinful, what are they?**
- **Do you view overeating as an issue of the heart or do you think labeling it as sin is an attempt to "fat shame"?**
- **What's the alternative to not acknowledging it as sin? See Prov. 29:1 Prov. 1:20-33.**
- **What's the promise for those who view it as sin and seek to turn from it? Read Prov. 28:13, Isa. 55: 6-7.**
- **Compose a prayer asking God for help to overcome your sin. If you don't see overeating as sin, pray that God would make you open to be willing to see it as He does.**

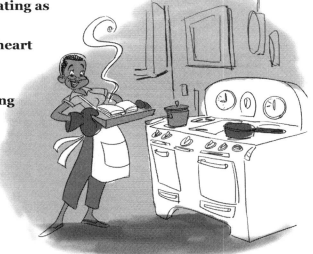

BECAUSE no one ever gained a pound from thinking too much.

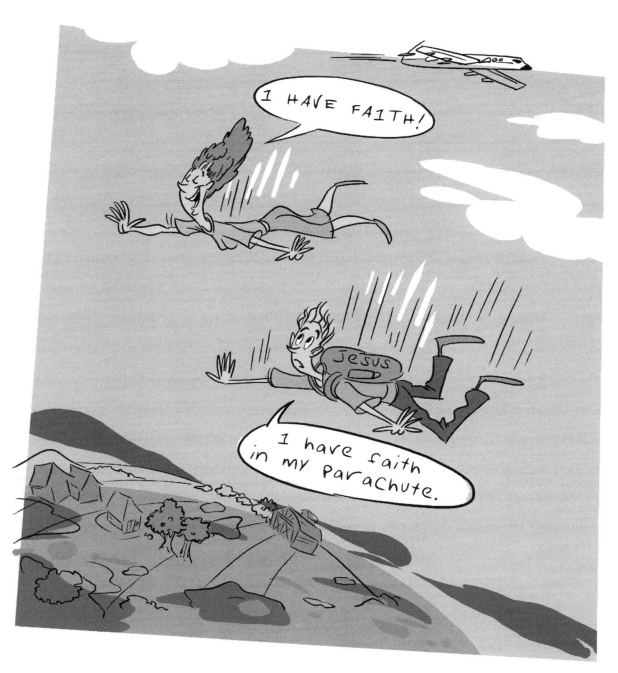

What's your faith in?

Chapter 6

# Who's Your Daddy?

> *For You light my lamp;*
> *The Lord my God illumines my darkness.*
> *For by You I can run upon a troop;*
> *And by my God I can leap over a wall.*
> Ps. 18:28–29

I used to be afraid of the dark, long after people should be. But eventually God gave me power over that fear so I'm no longer hindered by it.

Now heights . . .

Oh, yeah . . .

Heights *and* mountain lions. Terrified of them.

Which really isn't a problem—heights and mountain lions—if you're not in the mountains. I mean seriously, when's the last time a person fell to her death after being mauled by a mountain lion, while stuffing her face in front of the fridge in her kitchen? But everything changed after I started losing weight and discovered a love for hiking. So that's how I found myself, after midnight, trudging into the San Gabriels to view the "blood moon" lunar eclipse with a group of strangers I'd just met on the Internet.

Hey! At least I had my flashlight . . . and a man I didn't know from the group walking really, really fast in front of me.

As we returned from viewing the eclipse I discovered, to my dismay, that my flashlight was dimming. Yes, I had replacement batteries, but I couldn't get the stranger in front of me to pause long enough for me to change them. So I hurriedly tried to keep up with him in the dimming light of the night. At one point I almost walked off the ridge because I could barely see where the path had fallen away.

From there I clung to the wall in sheer terror and utter awkwardness as I tripped over the rocks that were next to the mountain face beside me.

I had all the right clothes, and enough water to make it the seven miles there and back, but without the right light, I was going to be destroyed. "Jesus please let me get home. Please let me get home," I whimpered, near tears.

After several minutes of silent terror, the man in front of me stopped, reached into his backpack, handed me his second flashlight, gave me some gruff instructions on how to use it, and then headed off into the darkness. What a difference! The path was just as rocky and dangerous, but at least now I could see it to navigate it safely.

I thought, as I came down that hill, *such is life.* There are pitfalls that happen to us all, and we're tempted to stumble around in fear and even blame God for our circumstances. Instead, we should be thanking Him for providing light to help us navigate those trials. The Bible says, *"God is Light, and in Him there is no darkness at all"* (1 John 1:5). It also says His Word is a lamp to our feet (Ps. 119:105). Wouldn't it be smart of us to become better acquainted with Him so we're equipped to make it along the inevitable dark ridges we might face in our lives with more confidence?

In the previous chapters I've written about God's sacrificial love that made a way for us to join His family and how obeying Him will give us direction to battle our long-term weight gain. Now I want to encourage you that you need to put in concerted effort to grow in your understanding of God and His character so you can find encouragement as you face trials—without running to sin.

I can hear you almost wilting. *UGH, you're loading works upon works onto my back, and I can't even get to the gym!*

I know what I'm writing can be overwhelming if you don't know God, but let me encourage you: seeking to know and understand God's character and attributes will not only empower you to do all He commands, it will also help you persevere throughout this lifelong race. You need to grow in your understanding of God because it will give you insight into the reasons for His actions in your life and help you understand why He asks what He's asking of you. Knowing God gives you confidence that your life is not out of control in times of trial because God who controls everything has the power to handle each situation based on attributes of His character. The knowledge of who He is also gives you confidence and a unique purpose individual to yourself. To top it all off, knowing God gives you better direction in your prayer life so even if the answer is No, you still have peace.

I don't know what Paul was struggling with when he asked God to remove his thorn in the flesh (2 Cor. 12:7–10). I don't know if it was a wearying spiritual battle, a physical malady, or just a really, really annoying person on his ministry team. God's answer was not to give Paul immediate relief, but instead *grace.* The biblical definition of grace is "loving-kindness, favor . . . the merciful kindness by which God, exerting his holy influence upon souls, turns them to Christ, keeps, strengthens, increases them in Christian faith, knowledge, affection, and kindles them to the exercise of the Christian virtues."[11]  In essence, God's answer to Paul was that God would rather give Him an increased understanding of Him and His abilities than give Paul ease. And for Paul, *that gift was a trade-up!*

We need to be like Paul. That means not merely being satisfied with trying to pick, pick, pick out that thorn in our flesh that makes us eat. Our earthly bodies are temporary, but what we know about God will see us into eternity. Growing in the knowledge of God not only prepares us for eternity, it gives us hope in today. What makes us think we can defend ourselves from physical, mental and emotional attacks? Our armor is futile. Almighty God cares for His children; understanding who He is gives us hope as we rely on His unchangeable, strong nature instead of running to other people or to things like an extra-large pepperoni pizza with mushrooms, black olives and house Italian dressing on the side.

We can get a head start growing in our understanding of Him through reading the Bible. But we need to not just read it, but take into our hearts what it says about God's character. Our God is everything good, admirable, just and mighty. He knows everything to an infinite degree; He loves you. Wouldn't it make sense to grow in your understanding of who He is?

# Finding the Hero in the History

Practically, though, how do you find Him?

If we're going to learn about God, we need to go to the same source that tells us how to live, for it will tell us Whom to live for! If we want to learn about God we need to learn about His attributes as expressed in the Bible.

God is the hero of the Bible. The first words of the book are, *"In the beginning God…"*

There are many ways to study the Bible: they all work if you're seeking to gain understanding about God and not just amassing knowledge. Like diets, they won't work if you don't do them. You have to find something that works for you, and not just because someone you admire does it. We're unique people, so it's okay that we learn differently. If you have a Bible study method that works for you by all means do it! I tried various Bible study plans before I came up with something that worked for me. For all my bluster and wordiness, I'm a pretty simple person who's easily distracted if a study process gets too multi-layered. I have a Bible dictionary, a concordance and a lexicon. I got all those things because other people had them. However looking through them was confusing for me, so I decided to just put them back on the shelf.

---

[11]  Thayer's Greek Lexicon, Electronic database. Copyright © 2002, 2003, 2006, 2011 by Biblesoft, Inc. All rights reserved. Used by permission. BibleSoft.com

I thought to myself, *God saved me . . . what does He want me to know about Him?* Interestingly enough, I formed my Bible study process after reading a book about writing screenplays. Roughly paraphrased, the author said the first character on any page, stage or screen, is the hero. The story's point of view will be different depending on whom we see first. Therefore a story that opens with a cheetah prowling the plain hungrily looking for lunch until it sees a gnu at the river and pounces on it, is a totally different story from one that starts with a gnu peacefully drinking at the river when it's snatched from the water in a flurry of splashing and fear. Therefore, since the Bible starts with God, then that shows us that He's the hero, and He is the lens through which every account in the Bible is focused.

I heard in a sermon from a well-known pastor that he approaches Scripture agnostically, which doesn't mean he doesn't believe it; it means that he doesn't know. Then he can read it without presuppositions, lightly holding onto other notions he's heard taught about that passage in the past. In this way, he allows himself to learn what's in front of him without being prejudiced by the past. We need to come to our Bible study the same way. God is the infinite Almighty! We can never stop learning about Him. We can never say, "Well, I got that mastered!" God's character is so enormous that there's no earthly way we can think just because we've gained a tiny bit of light about Him that we've by any means gained the total understanding of God.

As we study the Bible to find God, that understanding will govern how we live. To that end of seeking to understand the hero who saved me, I started to ask myself these questions when I read the Bible:

1) What is the universal truth that's being taught here?
2) What does this say about the character of God?
3) What does what I'm reading mean to me? How should this attribute of God affect my life?

## 1) What is the universal truth that's being taught here?

This takes into account who wrote the book and to whom was it written and includes obvious observations such as, "This is the account of Abraham entertaining heavenly guests" or "Paul is addressing the Corinthian church on a series of questions they've asked him." Oftentimes we skip over what's right on the page in front of us because we start looking for deeper meanings. Also, remember that the Bible wasn't written with chapter headings, so sometimes the actual theme might extend beyond that chapter break.

Don't make the mistake of thinking that just because the book was written to a specific audience that its *principles* don't apply to you today. A lot of issues in our current world stem from that contention: "Well, the culture was different at that time and because today we see things a lot differently we can disregard those commands that go against *our* culture." The Bible is written so that *all* believers in any time period or place know the character of God and how He has interacted with humanity. Jesus' earthly ministry attests to this: Remember He walked among us as God incarnate thousands of years after "In the beginning, God"—in a culture that was quite different from Adam's. Yet as Jesus taught His crowds of listeners, He dispelled any thoughts that His message was anything different from what His Father had originally commanded (Matt. 5:17–18).

## 2) What does this say about the character of God?

God is a person (for want of a better term). He is a *unique being,* not just some guy like your next-door neighbor in his boxer shorts and robe getting the newspaper on Sunday morning. As I said before, the Bible is about Him. Therefore everything that happens in the pages of the Book points to His personality and how He interacts with people. The Holy Scriptures aren't an account of Abraham, Isaac and Jacob, but *the God* of Abraham, Isaac and Jacob, and this God is *our God, as well.*

Now although the Bible is a book about God, sometimes you might have to look really hard for what an account has to say about Him. Just keep remembering that *every* event in the Bible has something to say about God's character even if at times He doesn't seem to appear. Sometimes His silences speak the loudest of all; in His seeming silence, God hasn't abandoned the person in the account. Even the fact the story exists in the narrative shows something about God's character. Since the Bible is God's inspired word, delivered by His messengers (2 Tim 3:16–17), it's God who told those narrators the stories. If God told them the stories, that means that the Lord Almighty walked through those trying, seemingly silent, times with those believers who may have experienced His silence, but *never His abandonment.* In this they found their hope, and God includes those stories as a reminder that so can we.

## 3) What does what I'm reading mean to me?

*How should this attribute of God affect my life?* Of course I have an opinion about the meaning of what I'm reading. I ask the sometimes-hard questions such as, "Why, God, did you do the things you did here?" It's not because I want to challenge Him, but rather because I genuinely want to understand the fact that God is a God of love who sometimes relates to His people in ways that may seem not to support that idea.

It isn't often you meet someone whose will is the beginning and ending of the argument. Sometimes it's comforting and sometimes it's annoying to know that God's character is the final answer to the question. God knows our hearts already. We need not to be afraid to express our doubts to Him instead of thinking we can't express them so that we secretly harbor them. He can help us work through our doubts to see Him as a God of love. You think that

God, who can read our thoughts, doesn't know we're bent out of shape about something we perceive about Him?

This is the personal application part. If God is the main player on the stage of life as this movie of earth unfolds, then I'm just a cameo appearance. How can I find comfort in some aspect of God's character I've just learned about? How should that cause me to live in obedience to Him, and how can it help me live in an understanding way with others?

This way of studying the Bible is what worked for me, but it's not law. You need to find the way learning about God works for you. Just seek Him!

The pursuit of knowing God must be paramount in our lives. Otherwise, any attempt to obey His commands won't last. God is the reason I started dealing with the issues that caused my long-term weight gain, and the reason I pick up the baton when I fall off the wagon with an embarrassing splat. God. Not just *God in concept;* but God, the real being whom I am growing to understand as time passes. God is a real being, not just a list of dos and don'ts. Deepening your apprehension of who He is makes His commands and His punishments more logical. Every created thing owes its existence to Him, so wouldn't it stand to reason that *His will* would be that against which everything that happens on this earth is measured? In essence He's like an atomic clock that governs the true measure of time, not like my great-uncle's pocket watch that silently drops a second here or there until, by the time it needs rewinding, it's several minutes behind reality.

In spite of who God is, too often we have reduced Him to a list of two-dimensional concepts. Then we're so surprised when He reacts in ways beyond our cardboard, tiny-box views of Him. That's what makes God seem to us random and grumpy. By growing in our knowledge of His character, we can gradually come to understand and appreciate Him for who He is. We can also understand why our choices elicit the responses from Him that they do. A beautiful thing occurs when we seek to understand Him better: with a humbled hush, we find that in the midst of understanding God as God, we are beginning to comprehend how greatly He loves us.

When we truly seek to comprehend Him for ourselves, He'll continue to refine and build on each bit we learn about Him. He will grow us spiritually, and we will find our purpose. If we have purpose, then we won't have time to sit around and eat to comfort ourselves when things don't go the way we wanted them to. Instead, continually seeking to understand God, we will pick ourselves up, dust ourselves off from the latest disappointment, and say, "Well, glad YOU know what You're doing—so what's next?"

Seeking to understand God more and more for who He really is—this is the key to unlocking our individual usefulness in the church, and the antidote to the disappointments and bitterness we often encounter when faced with difficult circumstances. The benefit for us is we don't eat when we're emotionally twisted up in knots, because as we grow in our understanding of His character, we find fewer things about which to be twisted!

In the end, each person on this earth will stand before God alone. None of us will be able to use the excuse, "Well, so and so said this about you and so I took that as truth." No, each person will be responsible with what they did with what they knew about God—*if* they knew God at all (Matt. 7:21–23). This applies to Christians and non-Christians alike.

God promises that those who seek Him will find Him (Heb. 11:6). You've probably picked up this book (if you're not one of my family or friends), because you've decided to lose more than a couple of pounds. Through the pages of the earlier chapters you may have identified the source of your external consequence (being overweight) and through repentance, you may have removed the rock of sin, as it were, from the field of your heart. However, it's not enough to dredge up the boulder, you must also fill in the hole left behind by its removal. Only an infinite God can replace your beloved sin. Anything else won't last.

## Beyond Being Just God Geeks

*Then Moses said to God, "Behold, I am going to the sons of Israel, and I will say to them, 'The God of your fathers has sent me to you.' Now they may say to me, 'What is His name?' What shall I say to them?" God said to Moses, "I AM WHO I AM"; and He said, "Thus you shall say to the sons of Israel, 'I AM has sent me to you.'" Ex. 3:13–14*

I hope you understand that when I encourage you to grow in your understanding of God it's not so you have lots of head knowledge about Him. You need to grow in your understanding of God so He can become lovely to your heart. So many times though, we stop at just reading the words of the page, seeing what God does and moving on with our lives without actually letting that impact us in any meaningful way

If you've watched the animated films for the last three decades, you're familiar with my friend Glen Keane's work. He's been responsible for some of the more memorable characters in those films including Ariel, Aladdin, Beast, Pocahontas and Tarzan. When he retired from the company just two years short of his fortieth anniversary, it caused quite a stir in the animation community and I found myself trying to explain who he was to a couple of friends of mine who weren't familiar with his work. To demonstrate what he'd done, I scoured the Internet to find scenes people had posted, which I knew were some of Glen's finer work, and

[9] From Merriam-Webster's Collegiate® Dictionary, 11th Edition ©2015, Merriam-Webster, Inc. (www.Merriam-Webster.com).

assembled them so my friends would understand how great an animator he is.

An interesting thing happened to me; while I was viewing the scenes, I began to cry, not so much because Glen is such an amazing technician, but because I'd *forgotten* how amazing Glen is as an artist. The reason is this: Over the years that I've known him, he and I have mostly spoken of our relationships with Jesus Christ, only giving a brushing glance to our jobs. In our every encounter, Glen's personal view on the world as he saw it through the lens of Scripture was always such an encouragement to me. From my point of view, Glen's view of God had eclipsed his tremendous talent. Other people knew him as a great artist, and that he is, but they only knew the surface part of him: what he did for a living. Because they geeked out only on his tremendous talent, they missed out on who he really was.

I think we in the church do the same thing with God. We're content to know Him for what He does, but *who He is* becomes another matter. The reason is that we mistake what He does for who He is. You are more than a housewife who puts amazing meals on the table that are gobbled up without the acknowledgement of the love and skill that went into preparing them. You are more than the skilled doctor who must compassionately deliver a patient's cancer diagnosis. You may do those things but all the while being a complex and unique human being. You just happen to wipe poopy butts at certain times of the day, but that doesn't define you.

When we stop at seeing God for what He does rather than understanding Him for who He is, we are being self-centered. He becomes either our errand boy who gives us gifts or our whipping boy when He doesn't do what we demand. But being moved by the character of God is how you can go beyond being just a God geek to being a person in His inner circle. It also gives us a Rock to cling to when we face trials, and it helps us understand how to approach Him in prayer.

## Knowing God as the Anchor of Our Hope and the Answer to Our Prayers

Seeking to be like Him dispels all doubts that we don't have someone who's really invested in our lives, who's unique and justified in making all His demands, and who's capable of fulfilling all His promises (1 Thess. 5:4).

Oftentimes we're content to skim the pages of the Bible, grab a nibble of its spiritual goodness, close the book, move on with the rest of our day, but then wonder why we struggle so much with trusting God. We need to cultivate going beyond a casual observance of how God and His attributes actually apply to us. We have to be careful that we aren't content to merely read the Bible to see how people's lives in the past were affected, or flip through the Scriptures for simple behavior modification ideas. Though there's some benefit in doing both of those things, in the end, studying the Bible for the lessons you can learn by

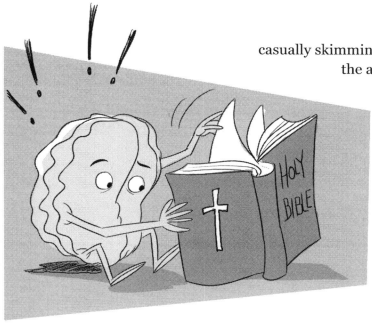

IS 10% of your brain only using 10 % of the bible?

casually skimming versus grappling with and applying the attributes of God to your life is the difference between eating a candy bar and a hearty meal before a seventeen-mile hike: one's going to get you a lot farther on your journey than the other.

God is more like diamonds than tree leaves. To know Him you must dig. I know the times I've grown the most are right after I've spent time in the word to learn who God is, rather than being content to only go to the Bible for how I should behave. There is a benefit in seeking Him that goes beyond being able to deal with our besetting sin. Seeking God in the quiet times of your life provides a confidence in Him during the desperate events that invariably befall us (Pss. 23; 27).

The Psalms adjure believers to seek the Lord. The interesting thing is that the psalmists don't tell believers to seek the Lord just because God will do stuff for them, they tell God's children to seek the Lord who will do stuff for them *because of who He is*. Each time in the Psalms where a person is commanded to seek the Lord, the charge is followed by attributes of God indicating why He's capable of coming to the aid of all who seek Him. One great example of this is Psalm 22, which is one of the ones Jesus quoted as He was dying. The psalmist who wrote the words was in anguish. However, he came to the conclusion that though there was great pain, there was also the promise that those who seek God will be able to praise Him. All of the words between the psalmist's anguished cries and that encouraging conclusion are a recitation of the attributes of God, which the psalmist applied as a salve to his broken heart. Jesus Himself models for us the benefits of seeking God, in that He was able to withstand His horrible torture and separation from His father by knowing God's character in advance (1 Pet 2:21–23).

In my times of seeking God for who He is instead of what He can do for me, I've often found the solutions I need. The bad behavior or life trial seems more likely to take care of it-self when I seek God. Understand that though I write all these things, I don't do them per-fectly. I go through seasons of gorging myself on God, then sadly follow them up with times of merely nibbling. I'm so glad God is patient with me—patient and resourceful. He won't let me stay spiritually hungry too long, eventually He drives me to a place where I realize He's the only answer to a trial He's sovereignly orchestrated in my life so that I, like Paul, run to Him and I am rewarded with His grace.

Not only does seeking to understand God help us in our desperation, it also helps us see more "Yes" answers to our prayers as well as respond rightly when He says, "No." *How does that work?* you may be asking. The Bible teaches that when a believer prays according to God's will He will answer their prayer (1 John 5:14–15). The best way to pray according to His will is not only to know His Word, but also to know who He is. There are so many grey areas in our lives, things that aren't necessarily covered in Scripture as "No" or "Yes". Should I take this job, marry this person, move to a house in the suburbs or a loft in the city? (I know, a lot of First World problems.) Knowing the character of God removes those grey areas. Likewise, since knowing who He is gives us clarity on what He prefers, learning about God's character will train us to be content when we hear "No" or "Wait" in answer to our prayers.

There will be times when we'll have greater problems in our lives than First World ones, and what we've learned by seeking God will give us the ability to trust Him as Christ was able to do on the cross while the world sneered and jeered Him and His Father temporarily turned His back on Him.

If only we'd look intently at the Bible and learn about God Himself we would see Someone so amazing, so unbelievable, Someone we're so unworthy of, that we'd become overwhelmed with the notion that this amazing God chooses to love us! God is Holy and yet He choose us to be with His children. As I stated before, He's like a parent who scrubs the dirt from his child who's been playing in the mud, all the while loving them for who they are beneath the dirt. All their quirks, talents, looks, and preferences—anything that's not tainted by the mud of sin—God wants it to shine through. In this we find our answer to "low self-esteem." We're not meant to think more highly of ourselves, but rather to understand and esteem God more highly. This is an unexpected grace. The gift of understanding the character of God is often not found because searching for God is such hard work, but it's a sacrifice worth making.

# Seeing God for Who He Really is Reveals Us As We Really Are

Before I finally surrendered to God and gave Him my appetite I saw Him as just the concept of God—Someone who'd win one day at the end of time and squish all His enemies. I was okay with that because I was on His team, but that's all I saw. Because of that, I secretly harbored doubts that He loved me and I thought following Him with unreserved abandon meant He would abolish my personality, everything that made me uniquely me. The way that I laughed, my non-sinful quirks, the way I viewed the world—poof! Gone. As I looked at the church I saw so many people who seemed the same as each other, and not like me. I was deeply, deeply lonely, but also profoundly afraid to lose myself.

What was wrong with me?

My view. What I was looking at. I was looking at the church and not looking at Him who was the head of it. I was looking to my brothers and sisters to define my identity, and not Him whose identity is so lovely I can't help but desire to reflect it. I was just a God geek: someone who appreciated the things God does, but who didn't really appreciate God for who He is. Because my concept of God was one-dimensional, of course I turned to people I could touch, who I thought were representations of my shallow understanding of Him.

God has given certain people to the church for the purpose of building the body (Eph. 4:11–13), but that doesn't mean you don't have a personal impact on the world around you by letting His likeness shine through you to the church and to your watching world (Eph. 4:15–16). We need to learn and grow from our teachers, but we also need to let the lessons we learn about God work through our unique lives.

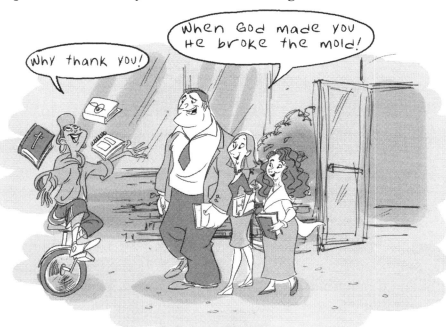

So many times, though, we stop our learning by scuffling our feet on the ground saying, "Who me? I'm nobody—I haven't got anything to offer, not like Sister Super Spiritual."

There's a theater game called "Mirror". To play it, a person stands across from a partner and they follow each other: leader follows follower; follower follows leader. It sounds pretty simple, but for some reason it is complicated, no sooner do you move your hand at the same time as the other person, and then tilt your head to imitate them, will you look down and notice their foot is raised and you missed when that happened. The solution is to look directly into the eyes of your partner. For some reason, looking into the eyes of your partner enables you to see the whole body.

The Bible likens the members of the church to a body with Christ as its head; it therefore admonishes the individual pieces of the body not to be bitter or disheartened because they aren't like another part of the body in function or attention. Instead the word of God instructs each of us in Christ's body, in a sense, not to follow the followers but instead to follow the leader. The answer is to look at Him who's the head (1 Cor. 12; Col. 1:15–20). As we look directly into the eyes of Him who saved us, we will discover how He works through each of us to accomplish His work in His way, with every single one of us as His resources.

As we begin to reflect on what His attributes specifically mean to us, our deepening understanding of Him affects our view of how we're made. As I saw glimpses of the beauty of God's character, I began to see my individuality in God. I saw that He had saved me, Carole Holliday, a creation for His pleasure and his purpose (Eph. 2:4–10). Focusing on the attributes of God shows up the foolish things we need to forsake for what they are. Only then can the beautiful things He created in us and wants to use us for come to light. That's when transformation can truly happen. It's not a change of our personality, but a true refining of our character.

So often we think we're not good enough because we aren't like those amazing Christians we're near. We forget that God created us purposefully with all our quirks and idiosyncrasies, and that whatever we do which isn't sin He loves, while whatever we do that is sin, He removes.

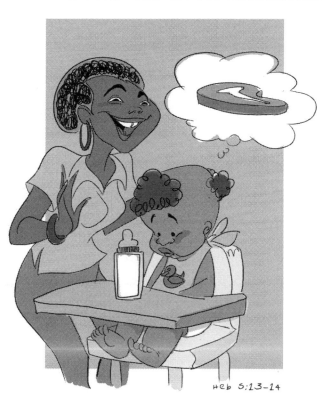

Heb 5:13–14

God is working in your life, just as He's working in the lives of those you admire, so instead of merely relying on their learning and example, strive to learn about God for yourself and you may one day find others looking to you because of your understanding of God. Then you can teach them to seek God for themselves!

While there's nothing wrong about admiring great things about others around you, when you admire them to the expense of your unique creation, then you're doing a disservice both to yourself and to the God who has a purpose for you that you alone can fulfill. Learning to see God for who He is gives you the ability to love yourself for who He made you.

So many times we fret as we search for God's will for our life and the answer is as plain as the nose on our face, or in this case, as the words on the pages of the Bible. Five years ago I decided to quit acting like a baby and feed myself the Bible: not because what others were teaching me was wrong, but simply because God said I could.

As I began to apply the things I was learning to my life, I had words to praise God when people asked me why and how I was losing the weight. A great deal of what I've learned about God is woven through the pages of this book. His holiness and love in particular have become hugely personal to me over the past five years as I've purposefully dealt with my sin and sought to understand Him better. When I began to express the things God was teaching me to others, people were encouraged. Eventually I saw that God was working through who I am and it had an impact on other people's lives. I was not even trying. I just wanted everyone to know how our amazing and marvelous God was revealing Himself to me.

As you seek to know God for yourself, you too will find ways to be God's evangel to the people around you—while just being you.

## Content with His Countenance

With all those benefits I've just unpacked regarding the cultivation of seeking to know God better, we still struggle to do it, in part because of two reasons: laziness and lack of contentment.

In Psalm 27:8 the psalmist said he would obey God and seek Him. In looking up the word "seek" in the Hebrew *(dârash),* I found that it means to inquire or resort to. It's interesting that it also means, "to frequent or tread a place." Think of the adorable image of a dog circling in one place before it lies down to sleep. Take note of the reason dogs do that: this instinct goes back to when they were wild and would have to tread down their surroundings to make a suitable place to sleep. Now dogs have cushions and carpets so their behavior looks silly. They don't need to make the ground soft because it's soft already. In today's Christian world, a great many of us have access to various sources of deep spiritual teaching, but sometimes we just rely on those instead of digging for the truths ourselves. I'm not saying all the books, commentaries, sermons and discussions we have with our friends are destructive; we need to make sure we're accurate in our understanding of God and so it helps to bounce our ideas off and learn from other saints. I'm just encouraging you to go deeper than staying there. We as humans need to return to the "canine past" and stop solely relying on the cushions and carpets of others' treading. We need to tread down our own beds. We don't seem to see that we're contenting ourselves to do the equivalent of sleeping on spiritual rocks, rather than treading a place in God by understanding Him for ourselves.

Other times, it's not the work involved in seeking God that puts us off, but our lack of contentment that makes us too frazzled, frustrated or unfocused to sit down and look for God who actually is the answer to all those issues that scramble our brains. Some of you truly are going through a trial, but a lot of us need to admit that we're just like cranky children who've been told they have to wait to have a cookie. When we're unable to come to peace with the situations in our lives as they are, we find that seeking God takes a back seat to the circumstances in our lives. How important it is to resist the temptation to pitch the very thing you need to help you get through your trial or crankiness—God's presence! So sit still in your trial. Sit still in your boredom. Sit still and know that He is God.

## Re-Educating the Robbers

I read a story recently about some criminals who'd broken into a shop and stolen all of the equipment only to return it with a note saying, "We had no idea what we were taking. Here's your stuff back. We hope that you guys can continue to make a difference in people's lives." The business they'd robbed provided counseling services for people who'd been victims of violent sexual abuse. While they were still criminals, the burglars returned the stolen property because they appreciated the character of those they'd robbed and they saw that it was good for their business to continue.

We think things might be easier if God just walked here with us, but look at Adam and Eve: They walked with Him and still they sinned. It's not enough to simply have God around casually; we have to grow to know Him for who He is. God is Holy. In various accounts in the Bible when people really got to know Him—I mean *really* saw Him for who He is—it brought them to their knees. They saw God for His amazing holiness and, not only that, but also their incredible sinfulness (Isa. 6:1–8; Luke 5:1–9; Acts 7:30–34; Heb. 12:18–29). As we learn more and more about Him, God gives us glimpses of that holiness, which helps us come to hate our sin and fight to overcome it and be ready to serve Him better.

In the end, it was seeing my sin of greed in the presence of God's holiness that lead me to repent of it. When I wander away, it's seeing God's holiness again that reminds me to repent, after it first brings me to my knees.

We share in God's likeness in some respects, but *remembering* isn't one of them. Because of our sinful, selfish bents, we forget God's kindness to us and, more sadly, we forget that He extended His kindness to us in order to save us from being destroyed by His holiness. We need to keep learning about Him to remind ourselves we are loved, and also to remember that the lover of our souls has saved us from His rightful and righteously justifiable destruction.

I'm wondering if this exhortation to study God might be pretty basic for some of you reading it. Why am I so insistent about it? All I can say is to offer my example. When God first convicted me that I needed to repent in the area of my appetite, I'd been a Christian for a long time. I'd gone to amazing churches with fabulous teaching. I knew tremendously godly people. Furthermore, I knew what *I thought* I knew about God. Even with all that in mind, I decided I needed to revisit and relearn the things I believed about Him so I could really get to know about God for myself. It was as if, after cleaning a cluttered room and after giving away the things I no longer needed and throwing away the things that could no longer be used, I finally had a clean space.

*Ahhh . . . That's nice . . .*

However after a while eventually junk mail found its way in. Something someone else didn't want ended up in my cupboard because they thought I'd like it. And so on. Eventually the clean space I once had was filled with little bits of clutter.

It's the same way with our view of God, if we're not careful. That little piece of the sermon we heard ten years ago by the pastor who's now changed his theology . . . that clever observation from our really godly friends that we have to remember . . . the tidbit we once read in the commentary . . . These things can be good, but at the same time they can also become clutter that stifles a growing view of God. God is infinite. We delude ourselves when we learn one thing about Him and let it fix Him in one place. We need to keep learning about Him, focusing on His attributes, and keeping our relationship with Him current; it's so much more than the things we've heard in the past.

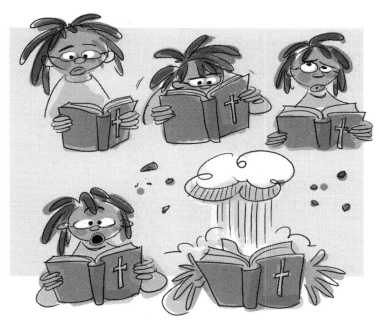

Mind. Blown.

If we want God's work to be revealed in our lives, we need to grow in our understanding of who He is. We think we can study long enough to understand some attribute of him and then be done with it. As if we think, *I know God; it's all good. Now I can go and watch my TV show.* God is enormous. He's more than enormous; He's infinite! Yet we think we can apprehend all of Him in a sitting? We're handicapping ourselves by being content to live on little scraps of God instead of continuously gorging ourselves on the understanding Him.

As you strive to overcome your greed or any other habitual sin, you'll find that your struggles decrease as you fill yourself with a knowledge of the God who created you. The character of God remains true even if you put your fingers in your ears and "la, la, la, la, la" all the way to the grave instead of seeking to understand Him more and more (Rom 3:3–4). He's like the fire in a hearth, which is warmer when you stand close to it, but which continues to be warm even when you move away from it. So cozy up to God and find the heat to thaw the cold places of your heart.

Even though it's hard work, we need to continually seek to know God who is the lover of our souls because doing so gives us the blessings of finding out who we really are in Him and gives us our purpose. Knowing Him helps us understand how to pray more effectively and helps us to be content in whatever God provides because we know His answers are based on His loving, all-knowing character. Not only that, as we learn about Him we learn what displeases Him, so we'll fight to avoid it. God in His holiness calls us to repent because His character is so pure He can't turn a blind eye to sin in His children.

God is a loving Father, but He's no sap. While He loves us for who we are, He won't tolerate our flagrant disregard for His holy character, commands and plans for the world for long.

· · · · · · · ·

*He who often thinks of God, will have a larger mind than the man who simply plods around this narrow globe. He may be a naturalist, boasting of his ability to dissect a beetle, anatomize a fly, or arrange insects and animals in classes with well nigh unutterable names; he may be a geologist, able to discourse of the megatherium and the plesiosaurus, and all kinds of extinct animals; he may imagine that his science, whatever it is, ennobles and enlarges his mind. I dare say it does, but after all, the most excellent study for expanding the soul, is the science of Christ, and him crucified, and the knowledge of the Godhead in the glorious Trinity. Nothing will so enlarge the intellect, nothing so magnify the whole soul of man, as a devout, earnest, continued investigation of the great subject of the Deity. And, whilst humbling and expanding, this subject is eminently consolatory. Oh, there is, in contemplating Christ, a balm for every wound; in musing on the Father, there is a quietus for every grief; and in the influence of the Holy Ghost, there is a balsam for every sore. Would you lose your sorrows? Would you drown your cares? Then go, plunge yourself in the Godhead's deepest sea; be lost in his immensity; and you shall come forth as from a couch of rest, refreshed and invigorated. I know nothing which can so comfort the soul; so calm the swelling billows of grief and sorrow; so speak peace to the winds of trial, as a devout musing upon the subject of the Godhead.* [12]

—*CH Spurgeon*

---

[12] Spurgeon, C.H, The Immutability of God, in The Surgeon Archive, http://www.spurgeon.org/sermons/0001.htm (accessed May 7, 2015).

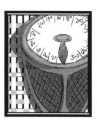

# Take A-Weigh

- Seek God for who He is, not just what He does for you.
- Knowing God will show you how to pray more effectively.
- Knowing God will help you find your own uniqueness.
- Knowing God helps you deal with your trials.
- Knowing God will cause you to turn from your sin.

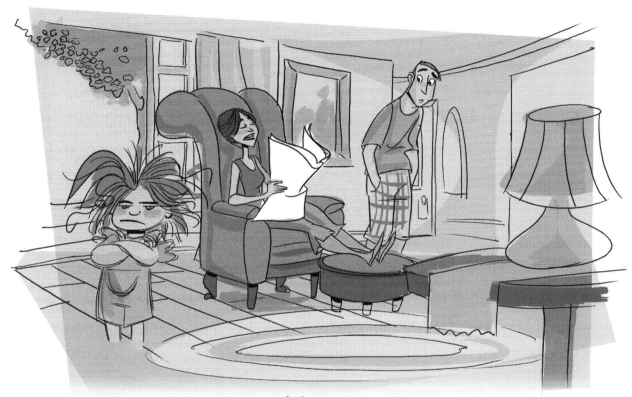

Don't. Ask.

## Chapter 7

# Tuck in Your Butts

> *It is for discipline that you endure; God deals with you as with sons; for what son is there whom his father does not discipline?*     Heb. 12:7

When my friend's daughter was about four, something the little girl did required she be disciplined. Though it was tough for the young mother to do, she took a small leather whacker, placed her little girl on her lap, explained her infraction and ended, giving the child a choice between two options: Say you're sorry or get a spank.

To my surprise, the little girl flattened her eyebrows, folded her arms and defiantly said, "Spankings." Was she insane? Did she think she was calling her mother's bluff? Who knows what went on in her tiny mind, but the little rebel got her wish.

Whack!

Her mother smacked her on her little bottom. It stung me to hear it but my friend, undeterred by my presence, looked her daughter in the eye and intoned.

"Say you're sorry."

"More spankings," the little girl growled in return. Her mother dutifully administered another sharp whack. The little girl didn't cry. She was too proud and angry for that.

This went on for five minutes. A slow, patient repetition of, "Say you're sorry" answered by the little girl's insistence she'd rather receive the whack than admit her wrong. Before long the little rebel's bottom glowed red and I marveled at her foolish pride.

Eventually the storm of rebellion passed and the little girl relented. "I'm sorry," she said in a voice of surrender. Her mother replied, "I forgive you." Then the little girl eagerly leaned toward her mother, lips pursed, where she was met with a willing kiss and a loving embrace. From there, the child scampered off, confident in her mother's love and protection.

In the last chapter I chose to focus on encouraging you to learn who God is for yourselves rather expounding on His specific attributes. The reason I made that choice is because there are plenty of super-learned theologians who are better equipped than I to explain God's attributes, due to their years of study and meditation. However I do want to touch lightly on one attribute of God as it applies to this book because it's the one attribute that convinced me it was time to change. It wasn't God's holiness, His love, or even His omnipotence; the attribute of God that caused me to eventually bow my knee was God's wrath that leads Him to discipline us.

God declares there are consequences for not obeying Him as both a powerful King and a loving Father. A king who rules his subjects without consequences won't remain a king very long. Likewise a father who parents his brood without consequences might as well be an abusive or absent dad for all the guidance he doesn't give his wayward children. As I mentioned in chapter 3 in the illustration of the disruptive child in the classroom, rebellious individuals would destroy themselves, while first throwing the world into chaos—without the wrath of God.

## The God Who Loves with More Spankings

What God wants most from us, is simply us. He wants control of our lives, our wills, our passions, and our pursuits. Yet often we complicate matters when we're faced with conforming our lives to God's will and we become like my friend's little girl with arms folded, eyebrows flattened, lips thin, insisting, "More spankings," rather than relenting.

I've seen this in my life: Before God gives me victory over some weak area of character, He first disciplines me, not only so I'll have the victory, but so I'll also have something greater—respect for Him because He not only disciplines me, but also guards and directs me

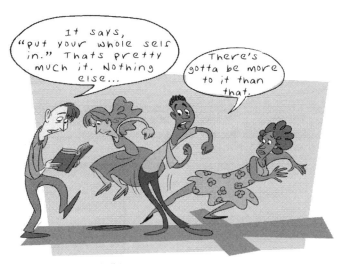

The simplicity of the Holy Hokey Pokey

(Ps. 119:73–77). In Psalm 23:4, King David said that God is the shepherd who holds both a rod and staff, which were a comfort to him. David, who had formerly been a shepherd, knew the practical uses of those tools. The shepherd's rod and staff protected the sheep from predators as well as correcting them when they were wayward. As I began to recognize God's rod and staff in my life, I started to see through the haze of my rebellion that God's relentless immutability in light of my pitiful assertion of will is not founded on His being petulant in anger, but on His perpetual love.

Because of the pain imposed on our stubborn wills, it may take a while to understand, *Oh wait, God's actually on my side,* but when we meditate on the discipline of our heavenly Father, we grow to love the hand that corrects because it protects us from both evils without as well as the wolves of personal sin within, which burn to savage our hearts (Jer. 17:9–10).

To see the love in the discipline of God, we must first embrace the concept of God's wrath. People don't like that word. Who am I kidding? I don't like that word. The word *wrath* makes me think of an enormous angry brute who's lashing out without reason or reasoning.

You're bristling. I know it. You're thinking, *I thought the Bible says "God is love." God can't get angry.*

But yes, God gets angry.

We think we're justified in demanding consequences when we're slighted, but God has to take it on the chin, smile and say, "Thanks for that. May I please have another?" Make no bones about it. God also gets angry. Since this is true, we need to understand the concept of His anger expressed through His wrath so we stop neutering Him and begin to grasp our sin's consequences.

## Rational, Justified Rage

The Bible says all creation points to the existence of God (Rom. 1:20). One thing to be learned from creation is there's always a center: From the universes that have one sun to the atom, which has one nucleus, and in between with man who has one brain. There's a central part that governs the workings of all. Yet we as humans are so presumptuous, thinking that we can be the brain, the sun, and the nucleus that drives the doings of the world.

The Bible also says that everything was created *for God* (Col. 1:1–17). When we realign our thinking, recognizing that the world doesn't revolve around us but that we're a part of a universe in which God's the center, we begin to see why He's justified when He expresses His wrath.

When we try to bend God to revolve around us and our plans rather than yield to His will, we're bound to experience tremendous friction. In cases such as these, God being God and us being human, guess which party comes up burned?

Basically speaking, because of who He is and what He's done, God is perfectly justified when He's angry about being wronged, and He has the power to do something about it. But He doesn't express His wrath without provocation. God Himself says the words in the Bible: "Vengeance is mine" (Deut. 32:35, quoted in Rom. 12:19). Yet His vengeance is always in *response* to something; vengeance is not something He initiates. In biblical instances of God's anger, He doesn't express it capriciously, but always in response to man's wrong against God. God who created the rules by which His world is governed has the right to judge and knows the exact punishment to suit the crime—from loss of love to loss of life eternal (Matt. 10:28).

That's why the Bible is here to give us the heads-up. God who says, "do this and live" is not just saying it so we have peace with one another on this earth, but so that ultimately we have peace with Him. The great marriages, healthy bodies, favor at work, and the ability to function capably are all just extras; peace with God is the prize. However, people don't see it that way.

Although people get bent out of shape because God wants them to live their lives according to what pleases Him, it's actually a kindness that He lets anyone know what He wants at all. Being God, He could be a big ole grump and just zap people with lightning bolts when they do something wrong so that others standing nearby might think, *Hmmm . . . Maybe I better not do that . . .* Instead, God is actually being incredibly kind when He tells us what makes Him angry through the Bible, so we'll avoid doing those things. However, our pride doesn't let us see this for the kindness it is; instead we see God's commands as unnecessary, random restrictions. But as I stated in chapter 3, God's commands aren't whims, but rather expressions of His character. So that's why all sin is against God Himself, even if it doesn't seem to have been directed at Him. From the tiniest "white lie" to the ungodly curse of a Satanist, whatever people do that counters God's standards makes them the center of the universe in their headstrong pride. Which is really silly if you come to think of it, because we're such finite and weak little creatures. The weak and finite, telling the infinite Almighty to go take a flying leap? Shudder . . .

This makes God angry.

It's hard to type those words, because I love the love of God. God's love is my hope in times of darkness and the reason I can change. It's also difficult for me to type these words because I know some of you're out there thinking, *Why should I follow God if He's going to get angry at me when I blow it? I might as well do my own thing!*

However, think about it. How's that working for you? Doing your own thing, getting divorced? Doing your own thing, getting high and losing all respectability? Doing your own thing and getting a disease from gluttony or sexual promiscuity?

Doing your own thing pretty much is what gets you into trouble. Even if there were no God to exact vengeance we'd do ourselves in, in pretty short order.

We need to stop thinking God's wrath makes Him some irrational bully who's tearing around the schoolyard indiscriminately picking on kids because He can. Instead we need to see He's a ruler who expresses His anger justifiably, as we too can do. Unlike us though, God is always right when He does it because He's completely fair and holds no favoritism (Deut. 10:17–18; Job 34:18–20; Luke 20:21; Rom. 2:4–12). He expresses His wrath both to those of high esteem and to those whom no one esteems at all.

We need to knock off God's-wrath-bashing. We need to quit softening the wrath of God as well; for seeing God as an angry God who exacts consequences on His enemies is the only way we can come to see Him as our only hope to *save* us from His wrath. Without understanding the wrath of God in its full fire, we miss grasping why Jesus' death on the cross was such a terrible and beautiful thing—in His death, Jesus, who's the embodiment of God's love, is also the One who satisfies the fire of God's wrath (1 John 4:10).

THAT'S where I truly saw God as love. Not the gushy, all warm, touchy-feely, earthly kind of love, but the jaw-dropping, knee-weakening, I-don't-deserve-this-one-bit at all kind.

This angry God, who had the right to destroy me because of my sin, instead poured the entire wrath reserved for me on His own Son, to pay for my sin. He didn't just forgive me; He gave someone else the penalty I deserved for the anger I incited. And God didn't stop there. After paying for my sin, He also gave me a righteousness that belongs to Him alone. Who deserves that much kindness? *No one.*

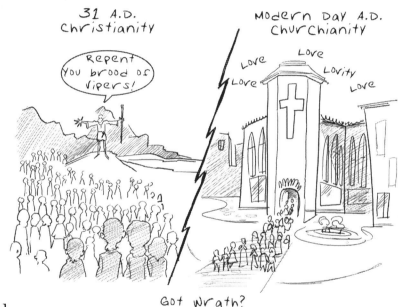

This brings tears to my eyes when I think of my willful depravity and God's willing love. I love the wrath of God because it always reminds me that God could destroy me, but by His own will and the work of Christ, He chooses not to.

Christians don't need to fear His wrath anymore because Christ has taken the nuclear bomb of His Father's retribution reserved for us. God has changed us from criminals to children and heirs. Anyone who has a child or has ever worked with one recognizes they need guidance to help them grow. The Bible says God's kindness leads us to repentance, but sometimes His kindness involves sharp discipline.

For the non-Christian, the wrath of God is a terrible and terrifying thing. There's nothing to save them from His wrath if they reject God's free gift of His crucified Son Jesus Christ. Non-Christians keep storing up His wrath until the day of judgment (Rom. 2:5–6), and believe you me, the broken relationships, messed-up health, lost jobs and property will be a cake walk compared to the eternal consequences that will be meted out to those who face the full blaze of His wrath when they finally stand before Him (Rom. 2:5–6). *Please, oh please, if you've made it this far in the book and are still unsaved: Run to God now to avoid having to pay the penalty yourself for inciting His wrath when you stand before Him after you die!*

For Christians, while we need no longer fear the wrath of God that leads to death, we don't get off scot-free from the consequences of displeasing Him. While we don't have to suffer the eternal consequence of our sin, God won't let us keep sinning wantonly. Instead He disciplines us, to make us stop.

God's discipline in the concerns of our daily lives serves a greater purpose than our daily lives, but just what is that greater purpose?

## When We're Sent to Stand in the Corner

Because God loves those He's saved, He disciplines them (Prov. 3:11–12; Rev. 3:19). There are different degrees of God's discipline in our lives.

I heard a parent tell a story of how he got his child to understand that touching the stove was hot. He first told him no, but when no didn't work, he smacked his hand and said "hot." Eventually, when the child still didn't get the message, the father allowed the child to touch the stove when he thought no one was looking, so that the child would learn firsthand the painful result of his rebellious decision.

This small story shows the different kinds of discipline God brings as a consequence to our sin:

- He tells us no.
- He openly punishes us.
- He allows us to suffer the pain.

*He tells us no.* Believe it or not, the admonition and direction of the Bible is a form of discipline. If you think about it, it's as sharp as a spank to your will to be told your way is not the right one (Ps. 50:16–17). God tells us No repeatedly through His Word; though it doesn't consist of: *You can't have any fun* but rather, *No, you will destroy yourself if you do that!* He does it not just so we'll live better lives; God disciplines us so we'll grow in our relationship with Him.

When we harbor a love for a pet sin, it causes us to be darkened in our understanding of Him (Eph. 4:17–24). Using my humble experience as an example: While I know I was saved all those years ago, the breadth of my understanding of God's character didn't expand until I finally began to repent of my greedy love of food and pursue sanctification in the area

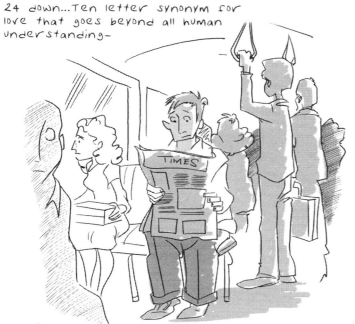

24 down...Ten letter synonym for love that goes beyond all human understanding—

but is commonly misunderstood...
Begins with a "D" and ends with an "e".

of my appetite. Seeing what I've gained, I'm ashamed it took me this long to trade my love of food for the love of the Father.

*He openly punishes us.* What if we don't respond to the gentle discipline of reading God's word? The next step in God's admonition to "knock it off" is to unleash the Holy Spirit, who's like an Australian shepherd dog in the pasture of our soul, nipping at the heels of our conscience.

One of the purposes of the Holy Spirit is to help us understand what God wants from us (John 14:26), so we can apply it to our lives. But when we don't act on what we understand, His admonition becomes more insistent. While a Christian is no longer under God's condemnation (Rom. 8:1), we still can feel God's conviction of our patterns of disobedience. It may come as a subtle twinge that comes when you're faced with temptation and Bible verses "pop" into your mind, or it may be that an actual thought occurs to you: *Hey, knucklehead! You're doing the wrong thing. Repent, right now!* Whether it's subtle or not-so-subtle, God is trying to get your attention to turn you from your sin. Sometimes at this point, He may also providentially send other people, sermons, books, or circumstances to correct you (Prov. 6:20–23; 19:20). Think how many times you have been in church and thought, *Wow, that sermon was aimed right at me!*

*He allows us to suffer the pain.* However if we continue to stick our fingers in our ears of our conscience, then God acts like the father with the child who insists on testing *why* the stove is no-man's-land. God disciplines His children with the consequences of their actions (Ps. 39:7–11; Prov. 1:20–33; Prov. 13:18; Prov. 15:10). This means that we are no longer shielded from ruined relationships, loss of status, loss of material goods, or even from loss of life. (Still, we remember Jesus promised in John 10:27-29 that nothing would snatch us from His hand.)

In this we learn the truth. God is God. Sin is bad. God is love.

Discipline is hard, but in the end, those who are truly His children will grow because of it. God disciplines His children because He loves them. Though it seems painful, it's actually the best for us in the long run. The Bible warns that fleeing from His reproof shows you despise yourself (Prov. 15:31–33).

What are some ways that God disciplines us when we refuse to listen to the teaching of His word; ignore the Holy Spirit's admonishments regarding our appetite; and proceed to live a lifestyle of unchecked greed, gluttony and covetousness? What are the consequences? Your relationship with God becomes weak, and you suffer from long-term weight gain. You incur all the biblical judgments pronounced on gluttons detailed in chapter 5, as well as condemnation from the people who see the evidence of your lack of self-restraint. God's final discipline can even be death. All these consequences in trade off for the habit of having that extra piece of pie . . .

That's the deception of sin: it feels good as it destroys you.

## Run From Your Razor Blades

My heart was broken when I heard a friend formerly was a self-cutter. When I asked her why she did it she said it was because it made her feel better. That kind of logic makes no sense to a right-thinking person, yet we who refuse to quit overeating do the same thing bodily as well as spiritually. We cut our souls when we sin in the false belief it will make us feel better. Every cut leaves a scar—on our conscience, our bodies, our minds, and on the testimony of our lives.

As someone who was in unrepentant greedy and covetous sin, I experienced all the forms of discipline: God insisted I repent, but I kept on sinning because it felt good. In addition to eating for entertainment, I was an emotional eater and sought to smother my problems by giving myself what my heart desired through my mouth rather than turning to God for His company, provision and comfort.

As far as God's discipline of me personally is concerned, I didn't know all the things I now know and have put in this book, but I did know that the Bible basically condemned greed and gluttony. I had many people warn me about the consequences of being overweight. I picked up books or heard things in sermons that pricked my conscience regarding self-control, but over time I began to be inured to the effects of God's discipline. I ignored the normal consequences to sin that were evident: health issues, being thought of as "less than" because I was fat and unattractive, and the occasional social embarrassment (like the time I was asked to move from an airplane emergency exit row seat because the stewardess thought I was too big to get through the door in the event of an emergency).

Ugh . . .

One of the darkest consequences (that still didn't arrest my course) was missing out on the final hours of my mother's life in ICU when she finally succumbed to cancer. I had come from work, eaten too much and was so uncomfortable by her bedside that I opted to go home to sleep away the discomfort of my binge. I reasoned I'd see her in the morning so I prayed with her, kissed her good night and left, not knowing I'd never see her this side of heaven again.

In my stubbornness and food lust, I was blind to see these consequences as anything more than normal results of making bad choices. I took a rather "meh" attitude toward them.

The Bible says Christians don't practice sin; yet, there I was getting really adroit at it. Though I didn't connect it at first, through it all I felt a dull and growing warning in my spirit: a subtle dread that my lack of obedience would be met with fatal force from a holy God who loved me, but who wouldn't continually condone my flagrant sin.

Yet my stupid pride would rather be beaten for the sake of "my precious," than to confess, forsake my sin and find forgiveness in the loving embrace and kiss of acceptance of my eternal Father. Why? Because I loved my sin—A LOT. I loved it more than I loved the God who created me.

But God relentlessly loved me too much to let me stay where I was (Heb. 12:4–12). Through His unyielding discipline, He eventually bent my will to His; I came to a point where it didn't matter if I lost the weight—I just wanted to obey Him and stop being greedy, because I finally understood that He is God.

Though the consequence for learning from God's discipline proved to be weight loss, confidence and many other benefits, those results were secondary to the blossoming of my relationship with Him.

In the end, God's discipline does more than give us better lives, it gives us what's best in life: God Himself. Obeying for the sake of pure obedience and seeing that as the end of your job as a Christian is as temporary as settling for the tin medal, half banana and quarter of orange they gave me at the half marathon finish line. God is the reward for all who run this oftentimes painful pride-crushing race toward the eventual winner's circle in eternity.

Through the unflinching discipline of His word, God builds our faith, transforms us into the image of Christ and trains our eyes to see God for Who He really is.

There's the moment when we are like the thief on the cross, who went from seeing Christ as someone to mock to understanding that Jesus was the innocent Messiah who could save him (Matt. 27:38–44; Luke 23:39–43). So many of us are content to live in that revelation of God only as a Savior, but God has so many more dimensions than that. If God gives us earthly life after we come to accept Him as Savior, surely it's because He wants us to know Him more fully than just as the rescuer of our souls. That understanding comes not just through dutifully cramming Bible verses into our heads and doing nothing with them, but by actively applying what we learn. As we release the things in the world that we love so much, God floods those emptied places with the light of the understanding of who He is. In this we come under His lordship, not slavishly fearing, but knowing that He loves us and we love Him in return by obeying His commands, especially in giving up our replacement gods.

Oh but how I wish that I had gotten the message to repent when God admonished me through His Word. Instead I was like the fat June bugs that throw themselves at the screen door of my house, repeatedly trying to go where they don't belong. I persisted in sinning so God was forced to keep stepping up the levels of discipline in my heart. Eventually, I stopped, not only because I want to avoid the pain, but because I longed to one day love God enough to stop without the extra discipline, just because He firmly told me to, and not because He had to spank me hard to do it.

## Hurried in the Wait

Another way God disciplines us is when He tells us to wait. While that seems like a strange form of discipline for a God who has the power over life and death to use, it can be just as effective as any form of chastisement.

God shows us in the discipline of the wait that He doesn't want us to be robots but He desires that we willingly dwell with Him in humble expectation of His work in the past, present, and in the future of our lives. In waiting, God gives us an opportunity to reflect on what He's done and our position before Him. Most times though, we miss the lessons we could be learning about ourselves in that quiet stretch between our perceived need and its fulfillment because we don't realize waiting *is the destination* of our life at that point.

When I moved to my town it was much smaller than it is today. One day I was in the mall and I was surprised to discover that the famed chef, Julia Child, was there to sign her latest book on baking. The air was electric as I hopped into the long line with the hope of getting her autograph on a book that I'd had no intention of buying until that moment. Everyone was buzzing with excitement. I spoke to the person in front of me and noted my astonishment at finding the renowned chef in my mall. He remarked that it surprised him even more, since "this town is only a pass-through between two bigger towns." His statement was funny, but well, it was also insulting. *Hey I live here!*

Oftentimes though, we're like that with God. We think our "waiting" isn't as important as where we've come from or where we're going. Yet in the small town of "waiting" is where we learn the greatest lesson. God is God (Ps. 46:10). If God's wrath shows us His displeasure, and God's discipline shows us how to be like Him, then our wait is when we see those things mix together to show God's rule.

God may seem to have forgotten us at those times, but He hasn't. The same God who rescued us from our hopeless, sinful state is the one who said to the nation of Israel that He was less likely to forget them than a mother would forget her nursing child (Isa. 49:14–16).

God is our Father who is in control over all things. Although He may put us in a time out, He doesn't forget about us while we're there. He's at work even while we are waiting because God's ultimate plan for our lives is to make us like Christ. God uses the time during our discipline of waiting to bring all circumstances to a transforming end in ways we can't even begin to comprehend.

So we need to submit to His discipline of waiting. I'm not saying this as though I've mastered it. I'm the queen of the spiritual eye roll when God disciplines me with a wait. I can often be like a teenager who's sulky that her plans have been changed by her parent. However, my sulkiness doesn't decrease the length of the time-out—often what it does instead is makes me remorseful once I've finished waiting, because I have not spent the time resting and preparing for what God had planned for me once He released me from the Land of Wait.

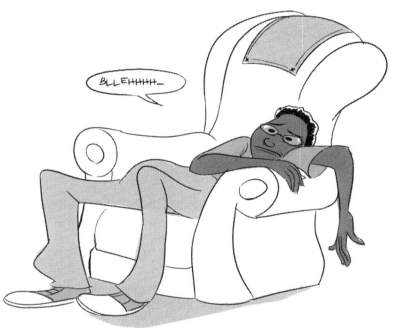

Yet the times I've submitted to waiting are the times where I've seen the most growth and accomplished the most work. It was when I couldn't find a job that I looked at my borderline-hoarder home and decided, *well, I guess I can take care of this mess* . . . then I took the next year of God's "wait" to work hard and put my house on a diet by going room by room, removing everything from it and returning only what was necessary. In a different season of God's "wait," while I longed for a more challenging job, I used the time to pursue exercising with more fervor than I would have if I'd been doing something more creative and mentally stimulating. In another instance, I used God's "wait" as I longed to be in a relationship with someone by taking all the insights gleaned while losing my weight to write *this book*. Most importantly, though, through all of this discipline of God's "waits," I deepened my understanding of the reality of Him.

We long to be in relationships with friends, or with an eventual spouse, or in positions of influence, or have more challenges in our lives. Those things may happen or they may not, but so often while we stand on the shore looking across the ocean to that faraway destination (whatever is our desired "paradise"), we miss the treasures we can pick up right at our feet that are found in learning about God and conscientiously addressing the sin He reveals in our lives.

So many times we hope God will intervene in our lives with some enormous supernatural act to give us grand purpose. While He does do that sometimes, I believe we miss out on the quieter displays of His power because we're too busy shouting over them, "Put me back in the game!" We miss out on the greatest changes He's working—the ones He works in our heart.

We need to stop viewing God's "waits" in our lives as something to merely endure. Instead we must understand that they're actual purposeful tools He's using to shape our characters for His glory.

I sing, but before I can perform, I must learn the music. In music notation, a composer indicates places where he or she wants the musicians and singers to rest with symbols on the sheet music. Some of the rests are little; barely time to catch a breath, while others are longer. If the performers blow through all of them, then the music is a cacophony instead of a song. Likewise in life, the cycles of rest and activity are widely seen and acknowledged (or if they're not, someone falls asleep at the wheel and crashes their car into an overpass). We need to look at the times of our wait as a rest even though it seems like a spank to our wills and our plans. When we do, God can fully equip us for what lies ahead.

## The Journey as Well as the Destination

As I wrote in my journal, *"God calls us to something more than just striving and self-determination. Just grinding along for the hope of better health only to be run over in a crosswalk by a bus while we jog.*

*"It's God, my spiritual* NORTH *on the compass of my life, who gives me hope even if all I long to accomplish falls flat. So what if I finish this goal: this last fifteen pounds and yet my eyes don't see the true 'NORTH' who is God? A job loss. A love unrequited. Something else completely unrelated to this journey to lose my weight, a zig in the road and I'm sent reeling. God wants to teach me to focus forward—to heaven where He, my real love, lives.*

*"I'm not comfortable with silence. I'm not comfortable with time. However those two things are where God deals with the hearts of man. That's where he deals with my heart. For the 'wait' is the time it takes for me to know His ways: like pausing for a moment after walking into the bright sunlight to let your eyes adjust so you can see what's there.*

*"When I run from the silence, when I try and speed up the time, that's when I fall. Even still . . . in the fall I see two things: one, that God forgives. and two, that God calls me to persevere. To get back in the car and drive not south to myself, but north to Him.*

*"The Christian life is as much about the drive as the destination. It's about the silent, monotonous road north. It isn't because God's cruel. There are just no shortcuts, and the*

*long way isn't just the long way; it's the right way. If He were cruel, then He wouldn't have paid the heavy toll to for me to be on this road in the first place.*

*"So what do I do? How do I mark time waiting to learn the lesson of the* NORTH *from a God who is outside of time?*

*"Just wait.*

*". . . and in the waiting, with an aching heart, cry out to the Lord.*

*" 'How long, oh Lord, how long? How long will it take until I get this lesson so that I see you?' My response to His answer determines where I am in the wait. For often I ask the question not so I can actually see Him, but so I can squirm on past this lesson to get to something I really want, like a child who chokes down the three brussels sprouts to get to the chocolate cake. But God knows. He knows the difference between the heart of a squirmer and the heart of a yearner.*

*"And I know He knows. And it frustrates me, because I can't get past the squirming… I don't even know how…*

*"Yet I have His promise in the wait . . .*

*I waited patiently for the Lord;*
*And He inclined to me and heard my cry.*
*He brought me up out of the pit of destruction, out of the miry clay,*
*And He set my feet upon a rock making my footsteps firm.*
*He put a new song in my mouth, a song of praise to our God;*
*Many will see and fear*
*And will trust in the Lord . . .*
*. . . Many, O Lord my God, are the wonders which You have done,*
*And Your thoughts toward us;*
*There is none to compare with You . . .*

*Ps. 40:1–3,5a*

*"God knows the time it takes to get me from point 'me' to point 'He'. He also knows the desire of my heart is for all those in my life to be inspired to turn over their pet sins as He has inspired me.*

*"And in this, I am caught up in His embrace and encouraged.*

*"Though the wait is still long and I still squirm; God, my God, showed me I also yearn."*

# Disciplined But Not Broken

If you're a non-Christian and you've made it this far through the book, then kudos to you! I hope that though you can see there's no getting around the wrath of God the choice is up to you as to which side of it do you want to find yourself: Is it the side where you pay the penalty for it yourself, or the side where you come to God for His forgiveness and then allow Him to lovingly teach and transform you through His discipline?

Ooh, ooh!!! I know—pick side B!

I hope you understand behind my lighthearted banter how much I sympathize with your struggle to come under God's discipline. It's a struggle only because we can't see the character of God clearly. So we fight, fuss and dig in our heels when we should lay down our arms and say, "Okay God, I surrender—open the eyes of my heart so I can see You and Your ways for what they really are."

The Bible tells how mankind should live with God and though it may seem harsh at times: in fact all God's commands are out of love (not only the commands with which we agree). In my pride, at first I didn't agree that eating less was good for me. It was my right, it felt good, it didn't hurt anyone, and it was just for me. One day that changed and God spanked my will so that I was forced to change. I could choose either God's mastery over my life or allow food to be my master. I chose God. Little did I know the very thing I thought was a simple decision would prove to be the beginning of my life! God was right. I was wrong.

So many people would say, "Duh, being fat is wrong. It's unhealthy and ugly." But God didn't say in the Bible, "Don't be fat." He said, "Don't be a glutton. Don't be greedy." The earth is full of people just like I was who will not agree with God that their particular set of sins is abhorrent. They too say, "I'm not hurting anyone, it's just me, and it's my right." Please hear my plea, though—God knows what's right for you. He loves you and His commands of discipline are for your eventual good. I've seen it to be true. For in obeying Him I went from, "If it feels good, do it," to "Oh my gosh, God, thank you! I didn't know how good it would feel to do what YOU said was good." All that started with belief in the sinless life, death and resurrection of Jesus Christ. He gives hope not just for eternity, but also for life right now.

God is justified in His wrath, but He spent it on His Son who willingly accepted it (Isa. 53:4–7). Those who stand in the shadow of the cross of Christ now experience not God's wrath, but His discipline. He disciplines us as the Bible says, like an earthy father who loves us. He's not the kind who strikes us out of anger. He doesn't tell us to quit crying or He'll give us something to really cry about. Nor is He a sappy, maudlin God-daddy who blubbers, "This is going to hurt me more than it hurts you …" God's compassion for us in our humanity expresses itself in His firm and unprejudiced discipline—because He loves us too much to leave us as we are (2 Pet. 3:8–9).

Sometimes He disciplines us with circumstances, sometimes with time-outs, but always through His word. In all those forms of discipline, He does it entirely from a heart of love with a desire to make us the best us we can be, because we're the "us" who are reflecting the image of Christ.

God makes it clear He doesn't want us to be "big-eyed greedy-guts," so we need to come under his discipline and prayerfully commit to repenting in this area. Take comfort in the thought that God isn't calling you to meet the world's standards of physical thinness. He's calling you to submit to His discipline and yield your control of everything to Him, even what you put in your mouth. Trust Him for the results in His due time as you live each day, each meal, each moment, in submission to Him.

Anything God disciplines you to turn away from, He equips you to do. He has too much invested in you already to leave you to deal with the monumental task of righting the capsized ship of your life by your own strength. In the next chapter we'll talk about the tools He gives each of His children to accomplish the repentance He creates in us through His discipline.

· · · · · · ·

*In the light of your personal holiness, interpret all the disciplinary dealings of God. All your trials, afflictions, bereavements, adversities, are sent as corrections of your heavenly Father but to promote your profit, that you might be a partaker of His holiness . . . "Then, Lord," you are ready to exclaim, "if this is the great end of Your discipline—if it be but to conform me to Your will, to expel sin from my heart, to imbue it with Your Spirit, and to mold me to Your Divine image, kindle the flame, fuel the furnace, use the flail, refine Your gold from the dross, and winnow Your wheat from the chaff- and let Your will, and not mine be done."* [13]

*Octavius Winslow*

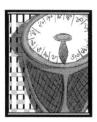

# Take A-Weigh

- God disciplines you because He loves you.
- God disciplines us through His Word, through His Spirit and through consequences.
- We need to obey the lessons He teaches us in discipline, regardless of our feelings.
- When God disciplines you with a time-out, learn all you can in that time so you'll be ready when He sends you into the next part of His plan for you.

---

[13] Octavius Winslow, *Our God* (London: John F. Shaw, 1870). Quoted at http://gracegems.org/WINSLOW/Our%20God.htm (accessed August 21, 2015).

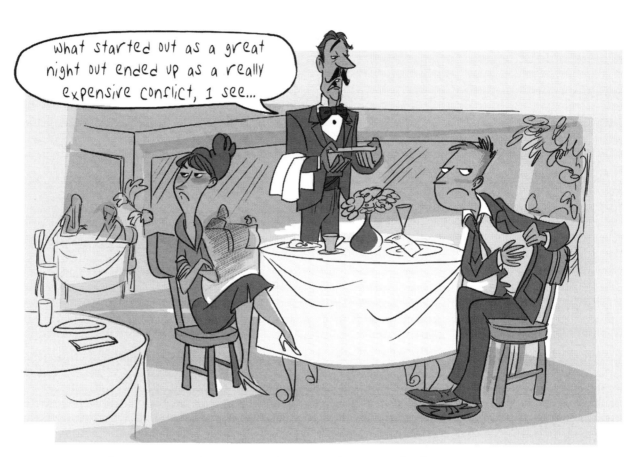

HE **NEEDED** the fruit of the spirit, what he got was humble pie.

# Chapter 8
# Walk This Way

*But I say, walk by the Spirit, and you will not carry out the desire of the flesh.*    *Gal. 5:16*

When I was a kid, one of the things I loved was getting the prize at the bottom of the box of cereal. By time I was in the fourth grade I'd figured out that I didn't have to wait to the end of the box to receive the plastic submarine powered by baking soda, or the decoder ring, or little plastic guy with the parachute that never deployed; I would just dump the box, get the prize and put the cereal back where it belonged. Then I'd forget about the cereal I actually first loved before there was even a prize in it.

Christians can be kind of guilty of that way of thinking. We want the prize of going to heaven, but often forget there's a whole bunch of healthy and nutritious cereal to sustain us through our day. Because we can't "dump the box" and just get the prize without waiting, we find ourselves frustrated, weak and powerless to live our daily lives. "If only we could just have the prize of heaven," we whimper, "then we wouldn't sin anymore!" But if we're still here and not in heaven, then it's for God's purpose, and because of that, He wants to make sure we're empowered to make it through the days of our lives. Because He's now our Father, He wants us to grow to look like Him so that we can be His testimony, representing Him before the world at large.

In the previous chapters we've looked at God's love, God's call and God's command to obey Him even down to giving up our most cherished sins. But we need to understand that He doesn't expect us to do what He asks all alone; God gives us a Helper to assist us in carrying out His commands.

The Holy Spirit, being the third person in the Trinity, has all the power of both the Father and Son. He is the guide to Christians (John 16:13). In sending us His Spirit, God makes sure that His children, who are fragile and unprotected from spiritual forces, the world, and sometimes even each other, are not truly alone. When Jesus returned to heaven He made sure we would have not only the power to survive, but also to flourish, that's why we are able to accomplish anything He commands us to undertake in regard to repentance.

So often we Christians look at the Holy Spirit the same way Bilbo from J.R.R. Tolkien's *The Hobbit* did when he first found the one ring to rule them all: To him it was just a ring at first, but later he would learn of its power. The power of the Holy Spirit gives us the ability to conquer all aspects of sin in our lives. With this gift, we don't have any excuse not to overcome our sin of greed except our own laziness. We need to stop keeping the Spirit in our mental pockets but remember to "slip Him on" and see what we can really do in Him!

Galatians 5:22–23 lists the ingredients in the cereal God gives us, and it's only by walking in the Spirit, who is our guide, that we'll be fortified to do all God commands. The ingredients of God's holy cereal are:

> *love*
> *joy*
> *peace*
> *patience*
> *kindness*
> *goodness*
> *faithfulness*
> *gentleness*
> *and self-control*

These make up the fruit of the Spirit. A friend of mine once said, "Carole, the Bible refers to the fruit of the Spirit, not the *fruits* of the Spirit. Singular, not plural as so many people mistakenly think. Meaning, if you have joy, you have peace. If you have gentleness you have patience, kindness, etc. If you don't have

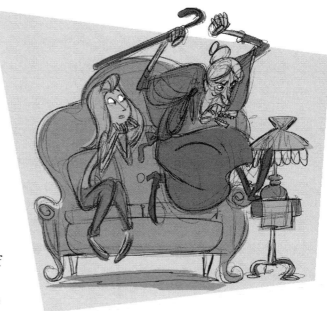

Patience doesn't always come with age.

self-control, for example—then maybe you don't have the Spirit, because you have all of them or none of them." That was pretty eye-opening for me. There was no way out of doing what God commanded with power—because everything I needed was already in my utility belt.

The statement did make me think; the fruit of the Spirit is a complete single package composed of segments like an orange. Some attributes of the fruit of the Spirit are harder to chew than others, but if you have some of it, you've got it all—although sometimes you have to work harder in your weaker areas. As my friend went on to say with a puckish smile, "The Bible says, 'Therefore I buffet my body to make it my slave . . .' Paul said buffet not *buffét* my body." So many times we should be pummeling our body but instead we're pampering it. The use of the fruit of the Spirit is powerful, but it's not magic. It actually takes exertion to use it.

The Greek definition for the word "fruit" in the case of Galatians 5 is "that which originates from." While it can refer to something like a banana or a kumquat, it's interesting that it also refers to progeny.

A man and woman can marry, make love and make a baby and the baby will look like them and never once come out looking like an alligator or orangutan. Likewise, the role of the Spirit in our life is to make sure we'll produce works that show we look like God and not the world. Godliness originates from Him, so it's going to manifest in us—as we walk in His power: *"But I say, walk by the Spirit, and you will not carry out the desire of the flesh"* (Gal. 5:16). The word for "walk" is *peripateite,* which means to make one's way, progress, to regulate one's life and to conduct one's self.[14]

We are being commanded to live our life in such a way as to constantly listen to the whispers of the Spirit as He speaks to our hearts. Our listening to those whispers gives the Spirit the opportunity to produce the fruit and do the things which transform us to look like our heavenly Father to all who see us.

This is why any of the godly attributes listed as fruit of the Spirit in a Christian are of a different stripe than those attributes as exercised by a non-Christian. Except for faithfulness, as we soon shall see in the context of this biblical list, Christians don't have a corner on self-control or any of the other named fruit of the Spirit. Plenty of admirable worldlings have demonstrated a level of mastery of these qualities in their lives, achieving success. For every beleaguered Christian who sacrifices the nicer things in life to support an ailing relative, there's a womanizing pro athlete who can be seen as equally generous for buying his mother a home from the proceeds of his multi-million-dollar sports contract.

The difference is to what end they're shown: for the glory of God. Our kindness or self-control or any of those attributes in the list is neither about us personally nor the people benefited by the expression of them through our lives, but *for God to display His work in us as He transforms us.* In the end, these are the only acts that will stand the test before God: not what we did, in a sense, but what we did *as empowered by Him.*

## Produce That Produces

So what exactly do those qualities mean? I know this may be basic for at least one of the two of you reading this book (though by now I've been assured that there will be at least five

---

[14] *Strong's Exhaustive Concordance,* #4043

people who want to read it, so I'm already up 200% in my readership) bear with me while I take a moment to explain each one briefly.

Paul introduced the fruit of the Spirit in his letter to the Galatians because he wanted to encourage his readers to remember it was only faith in the sacrificial death of Jesus Christ as a payment for their sinful nature that saved them. They were starting to think they needed to work to get God's delicious goodness. Once he'd set the record straight however, Paul knew their tendency would be to replace their legalistic lawfulness with libertine behavior thinking, *Well, since I'm saved by God's work alone, I can do whatever I darn well please and God will just look the other way, right?* Uhmm . . . No. Paul explains: It's not about doing good to get into God's good graces, it's about showing the evidence of God's total work, living as righteous examples of His transforming work in this world (Rom 6:1-7).

So the fruit of the Spirit isn't so that believers will have a better life—it's the evidence that God has made their life better already. Just as the smell of cookies baking in the oven does not precede the fact that the cookies are in the oven, the cookies produce the mouthwatering smell, and the Spirit produces the fruit.

*Love.* This one is the brotherly affection. It's different than what you feel for your significant other or your parents or even your cat. Brothers (and sisters) are people you're stuck with by birth. Sometimes you're more stuck than others, but you know they're in your life for good. The Bible tells us that through the Spirit, we will have the power to be bonded to one another the way we would be with our sibling, the one we may bicker with in private, but when someone comes along to pick on them, we'll throw off our hair weave and sock that person in the eye. The Spirit gives us kindredness that is useful for all kinds of things (I'll cover more about it in chapter 14).

*Joy.* We're not talking happiness based on circumstances, since those can change from moment to moment. Joy in a Christian springs from Whose we are and from the fact that we're Kingdom-bound. It comes in spite of the trials we face, as the Spirit reminds us that there's more to this life than the trials that beset us and even the blessings we find. There's something greater awaiting us in our eternal life and that should make us buzz with an underlying gladness (Rom. 14:17; 15:13; 1 Thess. 1:5–7).

*Peace.* This is tranquility with one another in the church, with our place in the world and, most importantly, with God. This peace is even more needful in light of the fact that often the message of the gospel of Christ actually brings discord because it points out people's sin (Matt. 10:34–38; Luke 12:49–53; John 14:26–27). The world gives prizes to peace-engendering people, but their concept of peace is only the horizontal kind: one person with another.

While that's fabulous, in the end it speaks nothing to the quiet unease of the soul in the night: . . . *Is all I've done enough to satisfy that higher something I can't exactly name?* The Holy Spirit assures those who are saved that God is no longer angry with them to the point of judgment. Though, as I said in the previous chapter, He may discipline them, He'll never condemn them. The Holy Spirit assures us we have the peace with God that no matter what happens in this momentary life (as compared to eternity) we will always have a place of acceptance in God's kingdom.

*Patience.* This is long-suffering endurance, steadfastness and slowness at avenging wrong. Godly patience is needful in trials that we face both from outside of the church as well as the conflicts we encounter with brothers and sisters in the family of Christ (2 Cor. 6:1–10; Col. 1:9–12). God knows it takes time for His children to have some light bulbs come on— some areas can be darkened longer than others. He's incredibly patient and kind with His children in order that they come to repentance. God shares that patience with us so that we can extend the same grace to others in the body. In this patience we strive to be like Him despite our contentions with one another. When we exhibit godly patience, we can become spiritual mommas and papas to people who are weaker in their understanding and implementation of God's commands. Likewise we can show graciousness of heart when our peers wound us with their sin "that they ought to know better than that to do".

*Kindness.* This is a specific type of kindness. It's a benign type, and it speaks of a quality of kindness and gentleness that's borne out of moral goodness and integrity. Growing in our understanding of God should produce not condescending pride but kindly humility. This goes far beyond the kindness of the womanizing B-baller who buys his mother a home, because the expression of his kindness, tainted by his immorality, comes from a sense of duty or because his mom is lovable. Spirit-produced kindness manifests in us a willingness to reach out to a person with whom we might struggle, or to act for the sake of others in a circumstance where we would normally want to be self-protecting. This kindness is self-sacrificial, which counters our human nature. God set His favor on us not because we deserved it, but because He was kind to do it (Eph. 2:1–7; Titus 3:3–7), and in this respect the Holy Spirit helps us to look like God. God whispers to our heart that our choices to act shouldn't be based on deservedness of the receiver or what we'd deem a "worthy" cause but our actions should be motivated on the need alone, and His love.

*Goodness.* This is uprightness of heart and life with some kindness thrown in (Eph. 5:8–10). While Christians can fall into temptation, can sin and can find forgiveness, the pattern of the life of a child of God is one that strives to be good. Think of someone who pole-vaults: everything they do is designed to get them over the pole. How they hold their hands, where they place them on the pole, where they place the pole in the ground, with what part of the body they lead, where they twist in the air and even at what time they know to let go of the pole. Sometimes they clear the bar, sometimes not, but it's the whole action that makes up the pole vaulting, not just clearing the bar. The better they learn to do all those actions, the more likely they are to clear that bar and even higher ones than that. Spirit-produced goodness *is the practice your life,* not just a singular act. The kindness aspect brings us back to the idea of that goodness working though humility. It's not enough to be "righteous" if you're not kind as well, otherwise you'll become a self-righteous punk that nobody likes, someone who drives people away from the Lord.

*Faithfulness.* This is the confidence that God exists and that Jesus is the Messiah. Outside of the church meaning, faithfulness means "being dependable," which is different from the faithfulness given by the Holy Spirit. The Spirit gives believers the conviction *that God is,* and that He has the ability to do everything He claims (thus validating His faithfulness in the sense of being trustworthy.) We put the cart before the horse to say God can do everything we think He can do. What we should understand first is, "who is this God person, anyway," and then we can learn what He's willing to do. Knowing and believing who God is first eliminates the presumptuousness of ginning up some demand, saying to God, "Anything I believe, you, God, have the power to achieve." Belief in God involves not only understanding His power, but also His principles and plans. Too many people have mistakenly tried to make God do what amounts to party tricks to satisfy their craven desires. It ought not to be that way with believers. We don't demand of God. We believe who God is and get in line with His plans.

I heard an analogy once that suits this definition: There was once a man who came upon another gentleman who was standing beside Niagara Falls with a wheelbarrow and a sign which read, "Tightrope Walk Today" The man was excited to see this feat and asked if the performer could really do what he'd promised. Without so much as a flicker of doubt, the acrobat hopped on the wire strung across the giant horseshoe-shaped falls and miraculously picked his way across the high-tension wire and back. Upon touching the ground to the thunderous applause of his audience of one, he asked, "Do you believe I can do it?" The onlooker having seen with his own eyes the skill of the man before him smiled broadly as he shook his head in the affirmative. "Then . . . " said the acrobat, grabbing the handles of the wheelbarrow, "Get in my barrow and let's go across together!"

We believe God raised His Son from the dead and we believe all the works Jesus did prior to that; we fully understanding what God is capable of doing. However, oftentimes we're loath to get in the wheelbarrow of obedience to His commands.

Faithfulness produces the ability to move forward through life based on God's character and in spite of what we can see with our eyes.

*Gentleness.* In a world where everyone is thumping their chests and interrupting one another to be first, the Spirit promotes meekness. God's gentleness may give us a mild disposition, but it doesn't make us docile lambs. We're more like tamed predatory cats. Deep down inside, each of us believes we have more to offer than at least someone else and yet the Spirit trains us to take what we know to be true about ourselves and to subordinate it to others. You cheer for the one who got the solo in the Christmas concert, when you thought you sang it better. Or you become the head of a ministry and serve the weakest people in it. Spirit-produced gentleness helps us be like Christ, the Creator, who willingly washed the dirty feet of twelve men—one of whom was going to betray Him.

*Self-Control.* With the fruit of self-control, you can master your desires and passions, particularly the ones that deals with your senses. A person who lacks self-control is someone who has cast off God's restraint and does whatever suits them (Phil. 3:18–19). It doesn't matter if anyone else gets hurt or is inconvenienced in the process. In the list of fruit, it's interesting: The one that deals specifically with ourselves is the last one mentioned. I wonder if, in the end, it's because even though all the fruit involves how we relate to the rest of the world around us, we still have to be the ones who take the reins of our desires in hand and compel ourselves to listen to the Spirit's exhortation to be loving, joyful, peaceful, patient, good, gentle and faithful.

We're our own greatest deterrents to the fruit of the Spirit being exhibited in our lives. We can say, "No thank you. I don't feel like being kind to Sister So-and-So; she's creepy." Or, "Hey, what do you mean I have to be patient with Pastor Fill-in-the-Blank, he ought to know better than to offend me. So what if he's only a flawed human; he's responsible to live everything he teaches perfectly!" Or, "No, I don't feel like being faithful because I'm super-tired. I had a horrible day and all I feel like doing is standing in front of the refrigerator and eating that gallon of ice cream, *before* I order two pizzas."

By giving us self-control, God makes sure we're without excuse when it comes to letting the good aroma of His work in our lives out to the world. Spirit-produced self-control helps us to not be the cork on that perfume bottle (2 Cor. 2:14–16). In fact, 2 Peter 1:2-11 indicates that self-control and other aspects of the fruit of the Spirit are marks of one's salvation.

Please don't get discouraged and think I'm saying that you're not saved if you're struggling in some area of sin because you aren't displaying self-control or any aspect of the fruit of the Sprit. Rather I want to encourage you: If you truly are a believer, you should step back and take a look at your arsenal and realize that you're not as helpless as you think.

God is the general of a giant battle, except His cavalry doesn't consist of nameless soldiers, but His very own children. He doesn't blithely put His very own heirs in the line of fire without equipping them to withstand the shelling from without and the arrows from within. He gives us the fruit of the Spirit to transform us day by day, not only to prepare us for His home, but also to battle on with increasing strength, as we remain alive on this earth.

## Stronger Than We Think

Through the process of understanding how my sin of greed affects my weight, I've come to see that the times I fail to eat like Christ are instances where I've not *used* the gift of His self-control, not that I don't *have* it. I acknowledge that I am the one making the choice to do wrong and not God, who has equipped me to behave rightly. I admit it's not easy to use those gifts because my "self" would rather be OUT of control and be self-gratifying. However as I struggle with each choice to come under God's discipline, I decide I love God more than myself, so that I am willing to do the hard work of using self-control to obey God in what I know is true: Quit being gluttonously greedy and eat less.

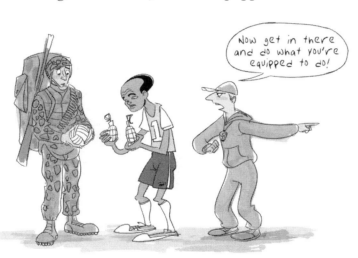

Now get in there and do what you're equipped to do!

God isn't like fallible man.
He'll always give us the right tools
to accomplish all His commands.

All Christians are given the fruit of the Spirit when we're saved. It's like being born with fingers and toes. Trying to perform any of God's commands is impossible without it. So many times though, we read any of God's commands and we think, "I don't have the patience for this . . . " or "I'm not self-controlled so I can't . . . " Well if what you're saying is true, then you're not a child of God. So realize it isn't that you don't have the ability if you're a true child of God; you may just be flat-out refusing to use what you've been given, or maybe you haven't learned to use your tool yet. Have you ever seen a baby run? They don't start out as Jesse Owens, but they do run. We as believers are given the fruit of the Spirit, but sometimes we need to grow in the use of it through practice.

Therefore by walking in the Spirit we approach all God's commands ignoring how we "feel" knowing our feelings are always going to make us decide to do nothing. We just do what God asks. If you fail to successfully navigate God's command for your life, as we so often do, ask for God's forgiveness. Take comfort in the fact that you're loved and forgiven. Then get up and continue to re-tackle that command, walking in the fruit you've been given. It's like when a teenager crashes the car and finds his parents are more concerned with his safety and teaching him to drive better than they are about punishing the teen for reaching for his taquitos when he should've had his eyes on the road. Remember that in the whole scheme of things, God doesn't discipline you for trying, failing, and trying again; He disciplines you for not trying at all.

When they fail to exhibit nonstop love, joy, peace, patience, kindness, goodness, faithfulness, gentleness and self-control, people often think, *Ugh, I don't have it . . . clearly I don't have enough faith.* (Well, at least I did.) Then we stay right were we have fallen. I hope you understand better now; if you're a believer, you DO have the power, but you're being a hypocrite when you act like you don't. You're just being lazy. Or, if you're not being lazy, then maybe it's because you're suffering from spiritual malnutrition. You can't expect to do God's stuff without God's constant companionship. You need to cultivate hearing His voice better so you can face choices to obey Him in your life in a manner that pleases Him.

I know the Bible speaks of the still small voice, but do you think the infinite God outside of the universe is content to be confined to a whisper? (Gen. 22:9–11; 1 Sam 3:2–9). We can amplify His voice by being in the Bible more. Right now I have a song playing on a loop in my brain because I heard it once on the Internet and decided to buy the album. The problem is that it's so catchy I find myself captive to the repeat button in my mind. It's pretty obnoxiously repetitious. Not only that, the thoughts of the things I did through the day, the good and the bad, my hopes and dreams for the future, all these things seek to muffle the small voice I should long to amplify. You and I live in a world of flesh and bone as we prepare for a Kingdom that our faith tells us will be made sight. God speaks to us through the Bible (2 Tim. 3:16–17). Just as we need to eat every so often to live, we need to feed purposefully on God's Word. Otherwise the songs and noise in our minds and in the world around us will pretty much drown Him out and we'll stall beside the path along the way home.

## Little Help From Your Huge Heavenly Friend

In chapter 6 I encouraged you to learn who God is, because understanding His character will help you toward your goal of being like Him as you strive against your sin. But I want to encourage you that there's another reason to learn who God is. A person who understands God's nature and abilities has the confidence to come to Him knowing what He has the power to do. That person also knows what God is willing to do. No one is going to go to a God they think is distant and not very powerful. What's the point if He's impotent or might be disinclined to listen? When you grow in your understanding of the truth of who God is, it dispels your doubts and builds your confidence to come to Him to ask what you need to obey Him.

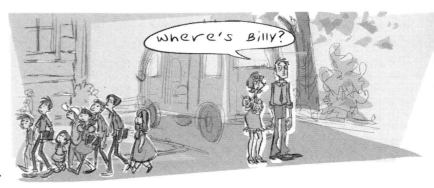

Not only does God give us the fruit of the Spirit to do all He asks of us, He gives us free access to come to Him for His comfort, His compassion and His power (Heb. 4:14–16). As I said in chapter 2, God doesn't give us birth and then leave us to do this thing called life on our own.

I haven't spent a lot of time focusing on prayer in the pages of this book as it affected my weight, because I almost forgot that I did it. I think that's how we often think of prayer. Like the fifth child in a family of ten who gets forgotten at church on occasion while the rest of them go home. Yet I did pray to God to change my life and give me the strength to obey His commands. I prayed for wisdom to help me come up with plans when I knew I was going to be put in a situation where I would face temptation (Matt. 6:13).

I'm ashamed to admit the other reason I neglected to mention prayer is because of my tiny faith. I prayed so many times as I've struggled to overcome this particular sin—and eventually I went ahead anyway, regardless of what I felt (which was generally nothing). Or if I felt something, it was that I was still afraid. When our feelings are unmoved in response to our prayers, it's easy to think that the results may have been our own, but that's not the case.

God works in ways we don't know regardless of our feelings or understanding, and just because we can't necessarily trace His hand plainly in a situation doesn't mean that He didn't orchestrate all the events and decisions in our lives to accomplish His divine answer to our prayers.

Remember that before God rescued Israel with mighty works, He first did the subtle, unseen job of hardening Pharaoh's heart (Ex. 9:12). I'm sure the Israelites would have preferred simply to be freed from their slavery in response to their praying instead of going through

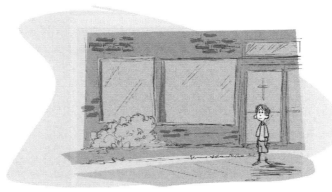

How come prayer often becomes like the fifth child out of ten that gets forgotten at church?

the cranky-Pharaoh stage, but if the Egyptians had just let them go without a hullabaloo then the Hebrews wouldn't have been able to see God work on their behalf to fulfill His four-hundred-year-old promise to Abraham so spectacularly.

Therefore never underestimate the way God answers your prayers and the time it takes Him to do it. Bear in mind that the way God answers them may not be only for you. In the case of Israel, He did all the things He did for them as an example for others down the line, like you and me when we read their story in the Bible (1 Cor. 10:1–11). As I look at His answers to my prayers in the course of losing this weight, I see that He has answered them in ways that may have helped me personally, but that in the end may prove to be a greater help to others as I share the lessons He taught me.

For example, my prayer to withstand the party with the cheese plate I love may not be seen as successful when I stand over it eating till I'm bursting. But God did answer that prayer by giving me a plan *for the next time I'm put in that same predicament*. In this, God teaches me bigger lessons. I learn how to be self-controlled, but I also learn that He's the giver of good gifts, even cheese, and He wants to give me the ability to enjoy those good gifts responsibly. God doesn't always answer our prayers the way we expect them to as we learn how to be like Him.

We need to come to God with hopeful expectation that He has a way to help us beyond any way we can imagine. If we're going to have any hope of finding the power to put down any sin in our lives we need to come to God for three things:

1. *We need to ask for His help.* Only proud people think they can get anywhere without stopping to ask for directions or refueling, yet we can be that kind of presumptuous about making our way to our heavenly home. I'm guilty of this. We have to remind ourselves that God has all the power in the universe and He's willing to share some with us to help us do what He calls us to do, whether it's from moving mountains in faith to moving our stubborn wills in repentance. God is ready to give us everything we need.

2. *We need to ask for His forgiveness when we fail.* One of the greatest deterrents to a relationship is being ashamed of our messes. Just think of the last time a friend surprised you with a visit and how reluctant you were to let them into your house because it was a mess. We can be like that with God when we have the mess of sin in our lives. Once we realize that we have sinned in some area, we can fall into the whole shame-to-guilt progression, which can put a wedge between God and us. Remember, God paid our entire penalty for our sin through Jesus so we never have to feel condemnation again—but we still need to ask for forgiveness. In that, we're simply acknowledging that we broke God's laws and deciding to try to avoid a repeat performance, and God readily forgives and cleanses us from our sin.

*3. We need to come to Him as He truly is.* A lot of times we come to God as though he's a distant dude on some far-off heavenly throne, or as though He's a big bad man with army boots ready to crush us like bugs. We have so many views of God that color our prayers when we come to Him that cause us to treat him in a way He doesn't deserve. Since our view of God motivates everything about our Christian walk I'm going to camp out here for a bit.

# Wash Your Hands Before You Come to the Table

In the time between when God left the Garden and when Jesus walked on the earth, He intermittently visited His people in the temple; however, only the chief priest for that year could enter into that place. Even then, there were all sorts of rules to govern how the priest was to enter the presence of God, lest he do so in an unclean manner and find himself without a job when he found himself without his life. However when Jesus walked the earth as the final priest mankind would ever need, He threw open the doors between God's holy presence and man's sinful world making it possible for any Tom, Dick, Harry, Letty, Jayne or Mary to come into His presence.

While God no longer strikes people dead for praying in an unclean way, He does hold to the idea that we must approach Him with holiness. I believe this is more than coming before Him confessing the sins that we know. While the Bible clearly warns that God will not hear the prayers of unsaved sinners (John 9:31; 1 Peter 3:12), we who are forgiven and paid for by the blood of Christ can nevertheless come before him in an unholy manner when we fail to talk to Him as He truly is. Treating something as holy means to treat it as sacred or hallowed, and Jesus taught His followers that God's very name was to be hallowed. (Matt. 6:9).

So often when I've approached God confessing my sins but forgetting who He is in His many facets and attributes, I wind up treating Him as if He were my heavenly genie instead of GOD. Sure, God has the power to answer all our prayers should He have the inclination to do so, and yes, we have the privilege (and command) through Christ to ask him for anything we need. But if we come before Him, list off our needs, and then toodle along our merry way without reverence to who He is, we are like the child with muddy feet who enters his mom's freshly mopped kitchen to grab a snack from the fridge, drink from the carton of juice, and wolf down her cake, leaving the cabinets and drawers open without so much as a "thank you." There's just so much disrespect in that scenario: too much to make up for on one Mother's Day a year. Still we do the same to God when we daily offer our "God gimmie prayers," only coming to Him with holy thoughts once a week on Sundays, thinking we're treating Him justly.

This is an exhortation to both myself and to you: Let's treat God as holy when we come before Him. We need to connect the things we learn about Him when we study His word to the way we approach Him, not so we'll have slavish fear but so we can come to Him as He is and find hope in the fact that He accepts us.

God longs for people who seek Him in spirit and in truth. I have been applying that to how we should come to Him as He created us uniquely to be, but it also applies to coming to Him in the truth of who HE is. Seeing God for who He is will change who we are when we reconcile His godly attributes with our sinful tendencies.

When Peter first met Jesus, he was on a boat, fishing. Jesus at that point was just a carpenter turned teacher. But the Lord presumed to tell Peter, a lifetime fisherman, how to do his job. Peter humored Jesus when he directed him to cast his nets on a particular side of the boat though they had been out all night and caught nothing. When he was rewarded for his obedience with a huge catch of fish, Peter didn't jump up and down and thank Jesus for the haul, instead he urged Jesus to, *"Go away from me Lord, for I am a sinful man!"* (Luke 5:1–10). Peter saw he had Jesus, who is holy, in his boat. Yet we are so blithe when we have Him in our houses, our cars, our walks in the park, or even in our hearts. We take God for granted because of His accessibility.

If you're not spending time reading your Bible, not only do you short-circuit your chances to learn how to look like Him, you also short-circuit your coming to Him as holy in prayer. For many years I approached Him in my flippant, unholy manner, rattling off my list of requests and satisfying myself that I'd spoken to the Creator of the Universe (which was the only one of His attributes I took the time to give a shallow acknowledgment of— and only that because I'm an artist). However as I've grown in my understanding of who He is, I have begun to grasp God as so much more, and that has changed how I approach Him. When I meditate on God's attributes learned in my studies, I am able to come to Him in a surrendered manner. While I am not the most excellent of pray-ers, the times when I have come to Him based on how He revealed Himself to me in His Word are the times when praying goes from commitment to communion. Sometimes this kind of prayer is a matter of discipline and takes quieting your soul, like putting down the fork when you've eaten to satisfaction.

## Getting to the Carnegie Hall of Prayers

"Excuse me sir, how do get to Carnegie Hall?"

"Practice, my boy . . . *Practice!*"

God knows we struggle to pray to Him in a right way, so just as the mother does not disown her son with the muddy feet, God doesn't strike us from heaven because we pray poorly. He may give us situations that help us to pray the way we should; He may encourage us in the example of others around us as we hear them pray emotionally raw and God-honoring prayers. Whatever way God grows us in our prayer life, we won't grow if we don't do it at all.

I had a piano teacher who wouldn't let me play if I made a mistake in the fingering. He would make me stop at the mistake, go back to the beginning and start again until I could play through that place. His premise was that he didn't want me to practice mistakes. The result, however, was that I was so frustrated by the process, I didn't want to play at all and eventually stopped. As a singer in my church choir, I'm one of the first ones to get the music memorized, not because I want to impress the choir director, but because I can't read music very well; I want to memorize the words quickly so I can look up and follow what the choir director wants from us. At first when I'm singing, I may not get the words quite right, but as I sing through the song with repetition, I hear where I mess up in relation to what others around me are singing and I remind myself mentally as I go along "I need to remember that," until eventually I have the song committed to heart.

God, our king and choir director, wants us to approach Him in the way he wrote the music we will one day sing in heaven: holy and reflective of Him. We're sure to stumble or get it wrong along the way. So while I'm exhorting us all to pray and approach God, remembering how holy He is, I'm also encouraging you to pray any way, even if it's imperfect. Start with praying to ask God to teach you how to pray. Jesus promised us that the Father in heaven will answer any prayer that we bring to Him that is according to His will. We know God will answer this prayer because the disciples asked Jesus the very same words: *"Lord, teach us to pray,"* and He did (Luke 11:1).

Above all, take a cue from the psalmists who prayed epic and raw heartfelt prayers beseeching God's help. Take time to be real before Him. He knows your heart anyway, so why try to be fancy? Talk to Him as you would talk to someone who is your only hope—because He is. Pray with honesty and trust He will empower you to accomplish everything He promised regarding your battling your sin.

Through it all, as you come to God remembering what His attributes are, remember above all to filter that knowledge of Him through the lens of understanding that He's your Father.

There's an iconic picture of President John F. Kennedy taken in 1963: he's sitting in the Oval office behind the Resolute desk shuffling some pages while his son John Jr. peeks out from underneath the desk through his "secret door to his house," as he called it. The three-year-old child didn't care that just the year before, his father had been in a tense standoff with the Russians on the brink of nuclear war during the Bay of Pigs, nor did the toddler know that in one month after the picture was taken, his father would be cut down by a disenfranchised man with a sniper's rifle during a happy little parade. All the little guy knew was that his father was his father, so armed with the understanding that he was loved and accepted by his daddy, little John-John was more than comfortable playing at the feet of the most powerful man in the free world.

*Our Father is infinitely powerful and He will never ever die . . .*

There are lots of books out there on how to pray so I won't belabor the specifics; I just want to encourage you to do it not only because we want God's Kingdom to come on earth, but also so He will make us ready to enter that Kingdom ourselves. I believe that if we treat prayer as though we are playing under God's Resolute desk then we'd find more joy in doing it. If we find joy in coming to Him who is more powerful than any great man in the universe, we will come to Him more often to find the help that we need.

So now you have all you need to get you going on the right track to obeying God, your choice now is do you want to move forward or not?

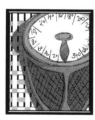

# Take A-Weigh

- The fruit of the Spirit is God's toolbox He's given for us to accomplish His commands in our lives.
- God also gives us power to battle our sin by praying.
- We need to join what we learn about Him to how we approach Him in prayer.

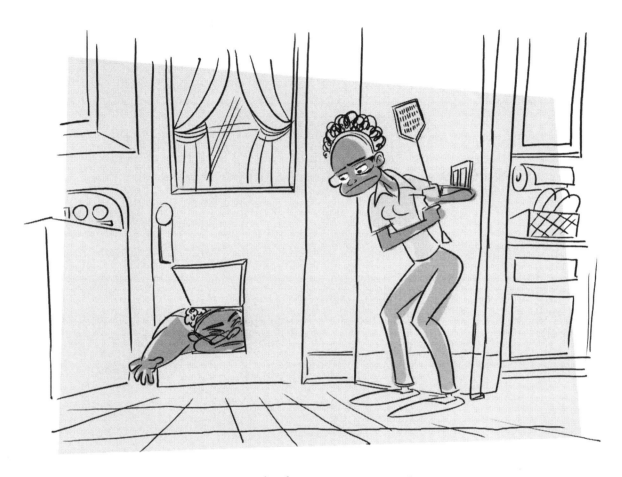

Make no provision for the flesh
Rom 13:14

Chapter 9

# You Mean I Have to Stop?

> *From that time Jesus began to preach and say, "Repent, for the kingdom of heaven is at hand."*    Matt. 4:17

I had climbed up there in the first place...

There I was clinging to a rock face about five stories above the hard desert floor, having just touched a carabiner pounded into the granite. Now I had to complete the task. The problem was that it meant letting go, falling back on the rope and letting my friend MJ guide me safely to the ground.... this same MJ who had convinced me to climb up there in the first place—me, who's afraid of heights. I trusted her because I knew her to be a dependable woman. I'd also seen her do the same feat she was asking me to do. And most importantly, I'd seen her safely belay other people earlier that day. It was scary, but I let go and fell, though I didn't do it perfectly. After a short, clumsy descent I gratefully touched the ground wearing my oh-so-awkward climbing harness.

Repentance can be like that. Oftentimes we've scaled so high in our practice of sin that returning to the ground of how God designed us to be is a daunting task—but we have to trust in the power of the One who is our belay, God Himself. We have to make a decision to do what God asks.

In the previous chapters I've written the *what* of everything God expects of the people He's given the privilege of adoption, but before the rubber hits the road and I address the *how* of dealing with the consequences of unchecked greed and gluttony, I want to gently encourage you as to *why* you should commit to fall in trust that God's often curious ways are the right ones. So often we come up with excuses not to repent and obey when we're convicted that we need to, like a little child at bedtime who asks for a glass of water, or to go potty, or one more story . . . We need to stop that if we're going to please God.

I've talked about the hope of the gospel, in that God sent His Son to die in the place of every man woman and child on this earth so we can be resurrected to the life we didn't

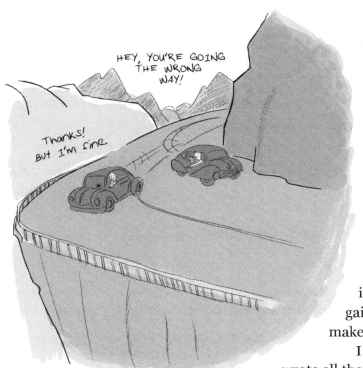

deserve. I've presented the knowledge that He makes us magically new so we CAN obey him from the heart so that His commands can cause us to look like Him. We've covered how no sin is more or less egregious to God, and how He disciplines His children to grow out of their sins and punishes nonbelievers to eternal death because of their rejection of His rule in their lives. I've encouraged you to get to know God, who gives each believer the power to overcome their sin, so that even if you are dealing with long-term weight gain, you can walk in God's commands and make your appetites His own.

I took the apostle Paul's approach as I wrote all these things, to give you hope as you seek to obey God and tackle this or any sin. Paul spent the first three chapters in the book of Ephesians extolling all the believers had in God through Jesus, summing up with his prayer that they would be strengthened by the Spirit and rooted in love, and that as a body they would really get a handle on just how much Jesus loves them (Eph. 3:14–19). I wrote about all these things because in the end, God's call to repentance and obedience is all about His love for us.

Repenting of a besetting sin like the one detailed in this book, is as much about turning away from those things that God calls rebellion as it is about turning TO God to learn that He provides better satisfaction than those sins do. Learning separated from turning won't produce lasting results. Just learning about God can make us become pompously self-righteous as we fill our minds with knowledge about a holy God but don't allow that increased understanding change how we live our lives. Just turning away from sin for the sake of "being good," can make us so tired that eventually we feel deprived and think life would be a bit more fun if we could only have a double loaded burger and two orders of fries instead of just one.

If we're saved, then we're in a relationship with God and that should affect every aspect of our lives, even how we approach turning away from our beloved sin. It elevates our repentance and obedience from only getting rid of actions and attitudes that produce inconvenient results to eliminating hindrances that interfere with our relationship with a loving God!

Bearing all that in mind, why is it sometimes so very difficult to repent, while other times it's so easy?

The simple answer is because we're stinkers and don't want to. There have been so many times when I can hear the words of God screaming in the ears of my heart: *Stop doing _____!* And I'm all, *Yeah, nope, not gonna happen.* I blast right ahead and do the very thing God hates.

My friend MJ commended me later for coming down from the wall, and I told her that was the only way I was going to get back, so what's to commend? She replied, "Yeah . . . but I've seen people take forever to make the decision to do it. One time a woman stayed up there for a half hour . . . " We may not want to give up our greed and gluttony, but we who are the children of God won't stay up on the granite wall of our beloved sin forever if we remember how much God loves us.

## The Tremendous Impact of Your Tiny Obediences

Every little choice we make has larger consequences than shrinking our waistlines.

As I've said several times in the course of this book: I don't think God cares what size you are. I don't think He cares if you're a ten or a double zero. He doesn't care if you look like a plain Jane or a supermodel with the best hair-do and a trendy wardrobe with fabulous makeup to match (1 Pet. 3:3–4).

But—

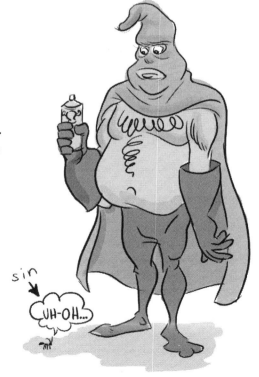

He does care about the sinful attitudes in your heart, which promote long-term weight gain, or make you slovenly, or late to work, or fill in the blank. He cares, and He lovingly presses forward, assiduously stamping out the secret sins buried in our hearts like an executioner stamping out the tiny sparks before they cause a firestorm.

The God who spoke the world into existence, from the greatest nebula to the tiniest atom, wants to put your life in order so that you can be with Him. Every command He gives us in the Bible is therefore not something to be checked off so you can say, "Okay, I've done that; what next?" No, you need to understand that God is not giving you a list of dos and don'ts, but rather leading you through the thorny paths of your wicked heart into the sunlight of His grace. Therefore, the things He tells you are not flat, disconnected commands; they are intricately thoughtful, loving pieces of a greater puzzle.

As you grasp this, it will help you avoid the temptation to pick and choose what to obey and what to ignore; you will understand the simple fact that, like the tiniest bits in a Tinkertoy® box, God's seemingly inconsequential commands are just as important to His ultimate purpose in your life as the big ones.

In other words, while God may not care how you look when you get to your weight loss goal, He does care about the food you put in your mouth as you seek to attain it.

At various points in my journey downward, I've thought of this passage of Scripture:

> *Whether, then, you eat or drink or whatever you do, do all to the glory of God. Give no offense either to Jews or to Greeks or to the church of God; just as I also please all men in all things, not seeking my own profit but the profit of the many, so that they may be saved.* 1 Cor. 10:31–33

This is a very powerful command to obey God to the point of killing my greedy over-indulgence. Yet if we look only at the part of the verse that applies to how we should approach sitting down to the dinner table, we miss God's greater goal in our appetite submission: His desire to show not only His love for us, but His overall love for mankind.

This is why your size, whether gargantuan because of your gluttony or skeletal because of your anorexia/bulimia, does have an impact on more than just you yourself. Your getting a handle on your appetite might be the only gospel tract your neighbor will ever see—or conversely, the very bomb that drives them further away from their gracious heavenly Father (Matt. 5:13–16; 1 Pet. 2:9–12; Rom. 2:17–24).

As I said in chapter 3, when we refuse to repent and obey regarding mastering our appetites, you and I demonstrate our practical atheism. By either our cavalier or our hyper-attentive attitude toward food we broadcast our subtle belief there's no God who judges the thoughts and intentions of the heart (Jer. 17:9–10), no imminent Ruler we'll one day face who'll demand an accounting of our lives (2 Cor. 5:9–10). Not only that, when we refuse to repent and obey we're also showing our selfish lack of love for our neighbors with our unspoken attitude of, *Well I got mine!* You figure you've got your in-ticket, bought for you irrevocably by the blood of Christ—so you erroneously believe you don't need to address the issue of working hard to eliminate the effects of your besetting sin of food worship, as it has shrouded you in layers of fat or overly exposed your frame.

Cast off your self-delusions and put on your big boy or big girl pants: Your appetite needs to be nailed to the cross—daily!

In your rebellion and laziness, you not only foolishly destroy yourself, you violate the two most important commandments in which all of God's commands are summed up: to love the Lord with all your heart, soul mind and strength and to love your neighbor as yourself.

So no, God doesn't care what size you are—but I guess in a sense He does.

I'm not going to lie to you; this journey down hasn't been an easy one for me. I'm torn as I intermittently wrestle with the reason why I overeat (I love food) and the fact that I understand people are watching. Ultimately though, those are the same reasons I press on to repent and obey what God has commanded of me. Even if I never make it to the magic weight loss number I've chosen in my head, I want to live my life in accordance to the prayer I meekly uttered when I first started:

"Lord, if I have one more day, one week, one year—let me live it to your glory."

That's why, when I stumble and fall regarding appetite control, I know I must always get back up. The "getting there" is not my end goal—it's the going. And going. And going—

To the glory of God's mysterious plan as yet to be revealed.

Do you see what your repentance and obedience actually communicates? Do you see that there aren't really ever any little acts, but every submission to God's will is important? Remind yourself of this always: It isn't for your weight loss that Jesus died, but for what put it on. This will help you repent and obey after your over-indulgence as soon as you realize you've fallen. Repent *right now* instead of waiting for tomorrow to begin again. Carry the importance of this with you as if your life depends on it.

## But Wait, I Don't Feel Like It...

> *Come, ye weary, heavy laden,*
> *Lost and ruined by the fall;*
> *If you tarry till you're better,*
> *You will never come at all:*
> *Not the righteous, not the righteous,*
> *Sinners Jesus came to call.* [15]
>     *— Joseph Hart*

You've experienced those occasions when you've sat on your leg wrong or put your arm in a strange position for a long time, and after you try and use that limb, you find it numb yet you force yourself to use it anyway—especially when you have to go to the bathroom. No dead leg is going to keep you from going potty because the consequences are less than desirable.

Yet often you and I say, "But I don't feel like obeying . . . " We wrinkle our backs with the idea of obedience. Since we're not robots how can God just expect us to say, *"Presto chango; I'm all repento!"* We fall into this resentment toward repentance because we think

---

[15] Hymn, "Come Ye Sinners," by Joseph Hart, lyrics 1759.

obedience begins with looking at God's Word and just doing what it says. This is a mechanical approach to obedience, and we're missing something extremely important when we do it. We're missing the relational aspect of God's commands. God doesn't want us to just do what He says because He told us so; remember He wants us to be like Him in the way a father delights to see his child maturing into his own likeness.

Therefore, when you see an area of your life that doesn't match God, your first response shouldn't be, *Hmmm . . . I have to come up with a plan to tackle this sin."* That won't suffice. No, we should come up with a plan to tackle our sin with a contrite heart that sees our unlikeness to God and longs to rectify that. Instead, pray, "God, I'm so sorry I'm not like you in this area. Please forgive me for my unlikeness to you. Help me to change so I look the way you say I should." Move forward, removing your feelings from the equation. It doesn't matter if you feel like obeying God. That's not the issue. Being like God is.

When Jesus called His followers to be perfect as His Father is perfect (Matt. 5:48), He had just detailed a whole list of commands that included rejoicing in the midst of persecution and loving their enemies—some pretty difficult things to do if they pivoted it on their feelings. Yet Christ was not urging their compliance motivated by their feelings, but rather because of the character of God, who is perfect.

I wish I could say I model this response perfectly when I'm faced with the choice to look like God without feeling like doing it. However God is faithful in spite of my faithlessness. He sits me on His lap and administers the discipline that brings me to the point of being willing to unfold my arms and be wrapped in His. After finding His forgiveness, transformation continues from there.

So start with acknowledging your sin of greed and move forward with the understanding God completely forgives you. Act like your Father in what He commands regardless of whether you feel like it or not. If you're struggling against God in any area, whether it's eating or any other sin, just make the first step—ask forgiveness—even if it's to say, "God forgive me, because I don't WANT to repent!" Make that confession and then walk in your Father's footsteps.

## Mis-Medicated Feelings

Christians get discouraged because they don't feel like obeying; they think they're not spiritually ready to repent. That's hogwash. Feelings have nothing to do with actions. Otherwise why would we ever get out of bed on Monday morning?

If we're honest with ourselves we actually do feel something when God calls us to repent and obey. That feeling is reluctance. We love how that sin makes us feel. We complain, "I'm bored, I'm lonely, I'm emotional . . . " and we sin in order to ameliorate those conditions. The sin makes us happy; it's self-gratifying. We're not looking so much for solutions to those negative feelings; we're just looking to feel good. Otherwise we would find something to do to combat the boredom, or call a friend so we're not alone, or actively trust God's sovereignty for the situations in our life that are making us emotional. What we're really thinking in those situations is "I like to eat a lot. It makes me happy."

Right now, for example, I want to eat though I'm not hungry. While I'd say it's because these book revisions are frustrating because they're taking forever and eating something would give me some satisfaction while I'm doing this burdensome task, in truth though, eating to placate a feeling serves only myself. The book revisions will still need to be finished. Even worse, if I continue to surrender to my appetite, I will disqualify myself from even being able to publish this book to encourage others (1 Cor. 9:25–26). We see in this example the sad effect of sin; though it promises comfort, in the end it provides only death (James 1:14–16).

We shouldn't let our feelings be the reason to obey or disbelieve God. As Christians, we came to Him in faith to be saved, not because we felt like it, but because God allowed us to see what terrible sinners we were and what a wonderful Savior He is. For my part, my initial feelings about the gravity of my sin in comparison to the holy Christ were so great that I was afraid He'd reject me. If I followed that feeling, I'd still be lost in my sin because I would have never come to Him for forgiveness. Would you have?

Furthermore, look at Jesus' example. He obeyed His Father despite His feelings. On the night before He was crucified Jesus struggled with feelings of anguish that wracked Him so desperately that He sweated drops of blood, and yet He chose to believe in His Father's plan rather than obey His feelings for self-preservation (Matt. 26; Mark 14; Luke 22). Imagine what despair the entire world would have faced had He chosen the opposite.

Quit waiting for your feelings: Obey God now. Every time you hesitate to obey because you don't feel like it, you slow down the advance of God's Kingdom, not only in your own life but also on this earth.

If you're a mature Christian who's struggling to obey you might rightly say that you need to ask God for power to do what He asks. The fine line to watch out for is that you might find yourself hung up on feelings again. *Okay, I asked God for power. Waiting to feel it . . .*

God's power is in His Word (Heb. 4:12). When you believe the Word to be true, already that shows that God's power is at work in you, for who would believe the words of a Being they've never seen unless that Being didn't first give them the power to believe in His existence? It follows that the power you ask for is laid in front of you simply by your doing what God asks you to do in the Bible. You have what you need to obey Him even when you don't feel like you do.

# The Engine is Running Even if You Can't Hear It

We also think we can't repent until we feel badly enough about our sin. Remember this: repentance means agreeing with God's will when it's different from yours and to stop doing your will and favor of His. That's all. Think of it this way: Do you have to feel badly before you will stop at a stoplight? Why not? Because you know the law of the land says red means stop. (And because you don't want to get T-boned by a car coming the other way.)

We think about how the sin affects only us. We think as long as we don't hurt anyone else with our personal greed, then what difference does it make if we eat one extra piece of pie or two? So when God says, "Don't eat that extra helping," it seems as if He does not love you but is randomly spoiling your good time. No, He's not. He hates your sin. So because of His love for you, He tells you not to do that sinful thing.

I have trained myself to think, *Eating this entire bag of chips right now may only affect me, but God, You say it's wrong. Because You've opened my eyes to see the sin that makes You angry, I'm going to put my trust in You and put this delicious bag away for another time.* (Or I may throw them away if I can't eat more than just a little.) When I choose to re-

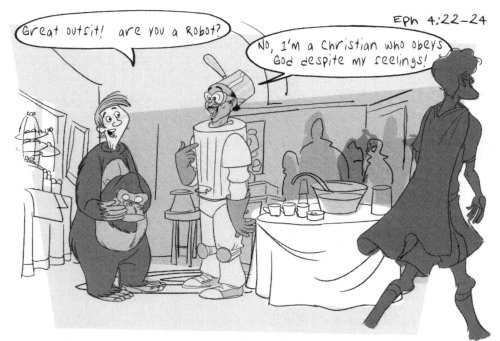

"...lay aside the old self, which is being corrupted in accordance with the lusts of deceit, and that you be renewed in the spirit of your mind, and PUT ON A NEW SELF, which in the likeness of God has been created in righteousness and holiness of the truth."          (emphasis mine.)

pent this way—when I do the thing that God tells me to do simply because He told me to do it—though it may seem robotic at first, eventually it shifts. In time, God's command doesn't sound like, "Do it because I told you so" but "Do it because I love you so."

More than ample feelings about repentance and obedience will follow.

So we commit to repent and obey by doing it. When we fail to obey, we repent and obey the next time. We're taking small steps with the long view in mind. It's something like potty-training a child. I don't have kids, but I've been told that the parent undertakes the hard work of teaching them to do the right thing in the right place because no one wants to still be changing poopy diapers when their son or daughter is thirty.

However, let me humbly remind you that if you're not saved, then this isn't for you. You'll be thinking you're doing God a favor by doing the right thing—if you think of God at all. Christians repent because the favor has already been done for them. They've had the lights turned on in the filthy room of their heart and then they gratefully start picking up the clutter according to God's directions. So if you're not saved, start with repenting of your disbelief in God and obey His invitation to come to Him for forgiveness. Confess your sins, believe in the death and resurrection of Jesus Christ and THEN you will have the power to repent because you will have been relocated to the Kingdom of Light. You'll have the power to belay down from that granite wall of your precious sin, even if it's scary hard, because you're held fast in the harness of God's love.

## Animating the Dustmen

Why do I encourage you to take this particular road to taming your appetite? Because in the end, all repentance comes back to demonstrating belief in God. As believers, we know our bodies are nothing but animated dust, and as we get older they get more decrepit and dustier. Far be it for me to add to what Paul said: *"Therefore we do not lose heart, but though our outer man is decaying, yet our inner man is being renewed day by day"* (2 Cor. 4:16).

Yet right before Paul wrote those words he also made an interesting statement: "I believed, therefore I spoke" (v. 13). Paul's belief caused him to speak. Imagine what would've happened if he hadn't believed. Or imagine what would've happened if he had believed yet didn't speak. What a horrible place we (who didn't meet Jesus miraculously on the Damascus road as Paul did) would be in: lost for all eternity (Acts 9:3–6; 15–16). The reason I want to encourage you to look to your eating habits is because how you eat is *an evidence of your belief, both to you yourself and the to world that sees you.* The world loses weight because they want to look good, feel good, get healthy or impress someone. As Christians, you and I are called to control our appetites to show that we're controlled by God. The bonus is we get all those things the world seeks—but along with an important gift—we already have the approval of the most important Person in the universe.

Understand that I'm not just encouraging you to repent and obey in order to lose that weight, I'm encouraging you to give God your appetites. Counter this world's drive: whose *"God is their appetite"* (Phil. 3:19). When you do this, your repentance and obedience to God's command to cease being a greedy glutton expresses your belief in God. Though this earthly body will be traded in for an upgraded model when you get to heaven, that doesn't mean that even these finite, squishy machines can't be used as a gospel tract to the watching world while we're still vertical.

When a poor unfortunate soul who's been adrift at sea with no hope of rescue, suddenly, against all odds, gets fished from the waters by a passing Coast Guard vessel, they have no end of details to share to all who'll listen, both of the terrors of waiting to die as well as the joy of being saved! Likewise, I want to tell everyone about the God who saved me from the penalty of my sin and who continues to save me from destructive actions. I saw in God's Word that greed is sin and He gave me the power to believe so that I stopped being greedy. He called for me to be His servant, and that steels my flesh for the long run and helps me resist food as my master. While I'm not perfect, I still point with confidence to His work shown in my life. Even when I fail, I have a platform to share about God's mercy, grace and forgiving love that leads me back to repentance. Yes, the King who rescued me is also devoted to see me through to standing before Him blameless with unreserved joy (Eph. 1:4).

Because my transformation is a result of choosing to repent of my ways and obey His commands in the Bible, I find I can extol the excellencies of God without being facetious and blithely saying, "Oh, God gave me the strength to do this." This also removes the idea that obedience is easy. While God does strengthen us, we also must work really, really hard (Phil. 2:12–13).

## Remaining in the Spotlight of His Grace

I know it's challenging to deny one's appetite—because we have to eat. It's so easy to slip over from "just enough" to "stuffing your face." It's not like drugs, where you just say no, or adultery, where you just don't hook up with someone to whom you're not married. We all have to eat. Some people can get away with overeating because their metabolisms work faster, so they don't suffer the consequences of long-term weight gain, but some of us can't hide our greed.

Paul warns the church in Ephesus not to sin in their anger so the devil wouldn't have a toehold—but there are many other ways we give Satan an opportunity to get his grubby little toes into our lives through unrepentant sin. However, the devil's toehold gives way in the face of repentance. Repentance blows the doors and windows of our hearts wide open so that God can clean out the shameful clutter and make us dwellings fit for the King. I praise God for my slow metabolism that rewarded my gluttony with a big behind and bloopy rolls of fat—I couldn't get away with it. I got to learn so many wonderful things about how much He loves me.

That's why I beg believers, thin or not, to consider the importance of repentance in the area of appetite. Eating right seems like such a small thing, but it's no small thing to do this small thing. Jesus said, *"He who is faithful in a very little thing is faithful also in much; and he who is unrighteous in a very little thing is unrighteous also in much"* (Luke 16:10). You never know; being faithful in this small thing may give you greater things for which to be faithful. In any case, you have the satisfaction of being a living sacrifice to the most High God, and what greater act of faithfulness can you ask for?

Overcoming gluttony alone is not the issue. Don't make the goal the weight lost, the marriage saved, the house cleaned, or the reputation restored, but make the goal of your life serving your God with your repentance and obedience. He will produce results when He desires. He has more invested in this than you do, having spent the blood of His precious Son to purchase you. He wants you to demonstrate *His work* in your life . . . not yours. Yes, it does require work on your part and you do have to eat less and move more, but the reason you do it is because of God. That's how I've persevered all this time in losing the

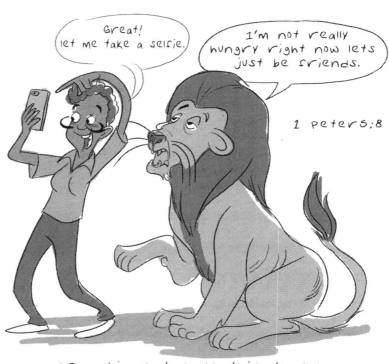

Great! let me take a selfie.

I'm not really hungry right now lets just be friends.

1 peters 5:8

If a big cat says this to you chances are he's lion.

weight and also in returning to the path of righteousness each time I've wandered from it. There's no summit to sanctification this side of death, just a continual climb toward Him.

Hopefully this takes the pressure off you. There is no time limit that HE puts on you: just day-by-day—no, meal-by-meal obedience. Though five years after starting, it's easier for me to do the right things now, it's still a battle at times to get out the door and go to the gym, or walk away from seconds . . . or thirds. Sigh. Yet as I pursue God's glory it becomes more consistent and not a fluke that I choose rightly.

As I write these words, I'm humbled at how much I need to remind myself constantly of them, because the longer I do this, the easier it is to slip into doing the good works because of the good results of looking good. Or I just plain get tired. I constantly need to recall Paul's warning to be careful how I stand (1 Cor. 10:12), lest I become like Robert Robinson, the writer of the hymn "Come Thou Fount of Every Blessing," who was purported to have fallen prey to the fears he wrote about:

> *Prone to wander, Lord, I feel it,*
> *Prone to leave the God I love*
> *Take my heart, O take and seal it*
> *Seal it for thy courts above.*[16]
>        —*Robert Robinson*

Long after the world's fanfare has died away because they're used to how we look, we'll always need to remind ourselves of these truths of the gospel of hope that transform us. For our hearts are always like wild beasts—smaller now, but still present—and our sinful desires will lash out when they can, with bacteria-tinged claws poised to spread infection to our souls. So we must always remind ourselves of the truths we have learned, just as God reminds me now through the writing of this book (2 Tim. 2:11–15).

## Doing What We Know and Not Just Knowing What to Do

Jesus demonstrated through the pattern of his life that obedience meant being God's willing servant and letting God be God. If Christ, being the Son of God, submitted Himself to the rules of His Father, we need to do the same. God left us His commands in the Bible as indications of His character working in our lives but we have to choose to act on what He teaches us (2 Tim. 3:16–17). James wrote that anyone who doesn't do what God reveals is foolish (James 2:20).

Therefore, if you know anything you're doing is wrong—stop doing it (Matt. 7:21–27).

Lighten the weight of obeying God's commands with the encouragement that it's actually a super-loving thing that God even tells us at all what He wants from us. So many times we work for or live with people who have rules that only they know. Like the time I was playing cribbage with a friend of mine and every now and again she would play something and then say, "Oh I forgot, you can go this way and get extra points for that." Which meant she was always in the lead, playing by her strangely unfolding revelation of the rules, and I was always going to be the loser.

God isn't like that. He gives us the whole rulebook in advance. He also takes into ac-

---

[16] Hymn, "Come Thou Fount," by Robert Robinson, lyrics 1757.

count we have teeny tiny amoeba brains compared to Him, and we can only remember His lessons from moment to moment. So He commands us to learn things through practice (John 3:21) and He looks at us through the lens of Jesus' perfection while we're stumbling through the learning process (Gal. 3:13–14).

That should bring us comfort, because in the end there's more to eating less than just eating less. By walking in obedience to something that seems mundane, we get closer to God.

Here's an analogy: When you got saved, it's as if you lived in the city where you could only see a star or two when you looked into the night sky. One of those stars was shining super-bright one night and you said, "Look, there's that special star—I want to go to there!" Though very few others could see that star, you started to make your way to it. However, being in the city with all its light pollution meant you couldn't see it very well, no matter how hard you strained your eyes. You had no car, but your desperate desire to see that star made you walk toward it. After many hours you finally reached the suburbs. There you could see the star a little better, but it was still not good enough—so you kept walking, and you went for miles and miles over days, crossing both rocky and flat terrain, past bogs, bugs and snakes to the empty desert. However, then you discovered that the entire sky is filled with stars! A pattern of obedience is like that. Eventually you will have the power to see more of the starry sky than you knew existed—because the Star has shown His existence to you (Eph. 5:14).

So get going and repent no matter how long it takes to see physical results. If you get frustrated with the length of time it takes to finish, I'll share something that helped me when I looked at how long it takes to lose the weight.

# Eating an Elephant One Bite at a Time

In the next chapter I'm going to tell you about some attitudes you will need to fight that have made you carry so much weight, but let me encourage you to face it all with an attitude of hope. Know that you can only do everything God calls you to do by pursuing your repentance and obedience *one moment at a time*. Otherwise, you'll become overwhelmed.

How does this look practically? I apply Jesus' command in Matthew 6:25–34 (to not worry about tomorrow, for today has enough concerns of its own) to our acts of repentance as well. There's a benefit to obeying just for today instead of being anxious about how we will have to fight the same difficult battle day after day; we pace ourselves. We make it harder on ourselves when we think of the long term. It's really kind of silly if you think about it: we're not guaranteed anything beyond the breath we just took, so why be anxious for results you may never see, worried about doing work we may not ever have to do? I constantly have to remind myself of this when I get discouraged thinking of the relentlessness cycle of repentance from greed.

When I live under the burden that I have to obey for all the tomorrows and not just today, I forget that though some days are tough, other days will not be so difficult. I forget that God will give me the grace to face my struggles as they come. Instead I fixate on the possibility that He will only always be silent so I learn to trust Him, but never have any relief in feeling His presence. Because I base my obedience on the bloody battle I just faced as I look at the future, I find it becomes easier to just give up under such weight. Have you faced this principle in dealing with some other relentless sin?

If so, then stop . . .

Did you know that your frustration and fear about the amount of time it takes to see results is presumptuous? It presumes you're going to be alive beyond lunch (Ps. 103:15–16). It presumes you're going to be alive beyond that act of repentance. Even now five years down the road, as I go through weeks of laser focus followed by weeks of indifferent laziness, I still have to remind myself of this.

Getting back on track, or on track in the first place, can be overwhelming. But we need to come to the realization that our repentance should be seen in light of our tenuous mortality and not in accomplishing our goal. Our seventy-plus years on earth isn't a guarantee; I could walk out my front door and get hit by a bus. So I need to repent and obey right now and not think about tomorrow. When I don't make the achievement of my goal my chief end, I find the pursuit of it easier . . . Okay, not easier—but at least not harder.

This seems like a bit of a contradiction. First I say we need to lose weight because the world sees our sin displayed in our long-term weight gain, but then I end with, "Don't worry about the results, but instead focus on each act of repentance and obedience in regard to your greed." Take encouragement that when you repent, you're actually doing the more difficult thing.

Remember, the world loses weight all the time, but only Christians are being transformed into the image of God. So actual under-the-hood repentance to get the car of weight loss running is more commendable than being able to slip into those size six skinny jeans. Think about what Jesus said to the paralytic: *"Your sins are forgiven"* (Matt. 9:1–8). The religious people around Him got bent out of shape at what they thought was His blasphemy. To which Christ replied, "Which is easier? To say your sins are forgiven or heal this person?" So to prove He had the authority to do the harder thing, He gave those detractors the external result: the man's physical healing.

Like that man, we too can be paralyzed, because long-term weight gain hinders our effectiveness in all aspects of our lives, but God has pronounced our sins are forgiven. Therefore though we still may look handicapped for a while by the consequences of our lives of willful rebellion, in our hearts we can walk freely. The weight we lose, though it may be difficult to achieve, is less impossible than removing the weight of our sin, which God has done. *So rejoice that you can even repent!* Focus on each act of obedience instead of the results gained from obeying and you'll get the results thrown in to boot!

Let me lighten your load so that you can focus on that one opportunity to obey your Father right now. Your holy, compassionate Father-King wants you to come to Him with each individual act of devotion as though it were precious. Each one acknowledges both His authority over you as well as your mortal fragility; your life is in His hands (Ps. 31:14–15).

So rejoice when you put down that fork as much, if not more, as when you lose that pound. Your act of repentance and obedience to the Lord brings Him joy, just as when a little child brings a small handful of wildflowers to his parent with a loving smile. The parent doesn't look at that child's meager offering of daisies, clutched in his pudgy little hand and reply, "Why didn't you bring me the entire field?" God the Father, who gave up His only begotten Son in order that we may become His children, doesn't sit there on the throne of grace when you bring to Him your broken, contrite heart and say, "That's all you have? Well that's not good enough. Bring it to me tomorrow and tomorrow and tomorrow."

Yes, we're called to live holy lives from the time we're saved as we prepare for our new home with Him, but we who are captives of time must live within its confines: as each moment in it. Your lifespan isn't in your hands, but what's right in front of you is. Focus on that moment, that action, and that one battle of your heart to eat right and bring to God your handful of daisies. Even if it's just one . . . then another and then another . . . Repent and eat in control now as though it were your last act before you closed your eyes on this mortal life. Though when you fade from this earth you may not be quite at your goal, because of the blood of Christ that cleanses you, God will be pleased with the beauty you've gained through your repentance (Phil. 1:6).

In due season each act of repentance and obedience will produce a gradual change beyond your smaller size.

## More Than Just the Thinner You

The Carole I am today is so different from Carole I was five years ago. Not just because I'm a smaller size and not because I'm some kind of amazing rock-star at obedience, because I still struggle. No, I'm not at my magic number, but as I think about it, my life looks different. I've found peace, hope, and joy in God, not despair and pressure to perform. I see that I have an amazing God who's incrementally transforming me in the most unique of ways. I've learned to see that when I have a problem with a command, it's not because it's a bad idea, but because I'm being a punk in not wanting to do it. I've learned to appreciate His firm love that gives me guidance and, when I've slipped up, His heavy hand of righteousness on my heart

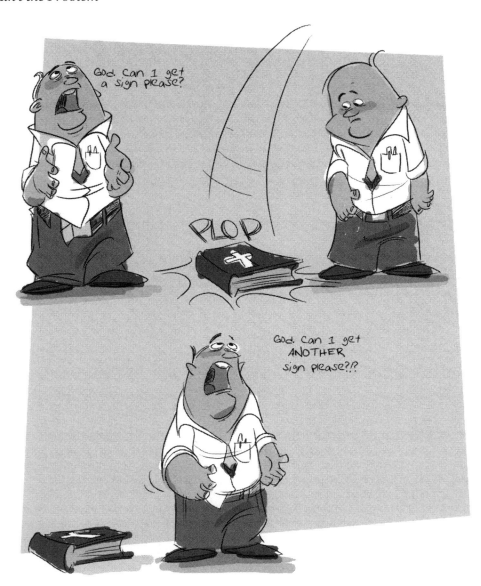

that kindly leads me to repent.

Above all, God has enlightened the eyes of my heart to see He's not a despotic ruler, but a loving Father, waiting to welcome His children home. The difference is more than a change in how I see Him; it's also a change in how I see myself, as well. God has given me a value as a person I never realized I could have in all the years I was stridently asserting my own individuality.

So often when people lose weight they find they gain a new sense of confidence. They learn to say no to things they don't like, instead of trying to please everyone (because they're no longer fat and have to get people to like them). They may become more or less in-your-face, or strident and assertive, as if they need to show the world, "Look what you missed out by shunning me. Nyah, Nyah!" However, if all you get from losing weight is better health and a shiny new sense of self-esteem, then you've settled for the bird in the hand when you could have God's treasure in the bush.

Our bodies, no matter how well we take care of them, will eventually fail, wrecked by time or some inherited disease. Our sense of confidence is incredibly fragile as it always seems to be based on comparison to others—no matter how hard we fight against it. So there's got to be something more.

God wants to give you that more, He wants to give you *you!*

You are, as Jesus works through you, amazing! There's no one like you. Don't you want to meet this person? Well you can, but only if you repent. If you cast off all these layers of sinful attitudes and actions, like when you shed a heavy coat when the winter day suddenly turns warm, you'll find both relief and show the world what's been hidden beneath those layers of sin you cherished.

So now you know. God calls us to repentance, but he doesn't leave us unequipped to do what he's asked. We have everything we need to obey Him from the heart if we just walk in it despite how we feel. When we do this, we grow to see how repenting of our greed isn't just about ourselves, but it's showing the world just how much God loves. So let go of your death grip on the granite wall of your sin, fall back and let God take you down to the safety of Him.

How does this look practically, in terms of actually purposing to lose your weight? Read on and you'll see how it worked practically in my life.

· · · · · · ·

*For this is the love of God, that we keep His commandments; and His commandments are not burdensome. For whatever is born of God overcomes the world; and this is the victory that has overcome the world—our faith. Who is the one who overcomes the world, but he who believes that Jesus is the Son of God?*     *1 John 5:3–5*

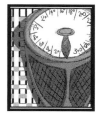

# Take A-Weigh

- Repentance and obedience proves God's existence to a watching world.
- Repentance and obedience needs to happen regardless of our feelings.
- Repentance and obedience is our way of life and not only for results.
- God asks for our repentance and obedience because He loves us.
- Repentance and obedience gives God the chance to show the world our real self.

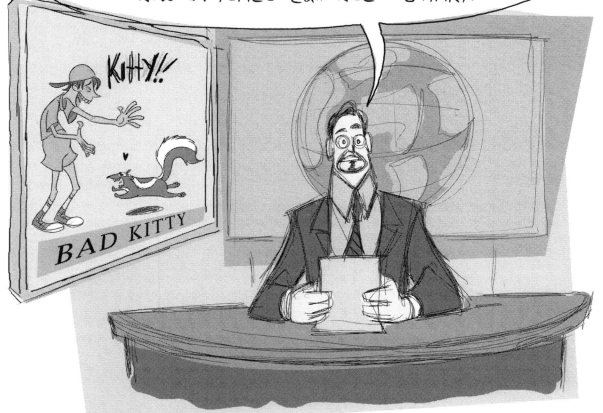

obey God and you wont Get skunked!

Chapter 10

# The Not Diet

> *Therefore I urge you, brethren, by the mercies of God, to present your bodies a living and holy sacrifice, acceptable to God, which is your spiritual service of worship. And do not be conformed to this world, but be transformed by the renewing of your mind, so that you may prove what the will of God is, that which is good and acceptable and perfect.* Romans 12:1–2

I mentioned my friend Carol already. She's the one with the really tall desk. She's also someone who's had a giant impact in my life.

Whenever we introduce ourselves we say, *"I'm Carole; she's Carol. I look like mom; she looks like dad."* Yes, while the obvious fact that she's white and I'm black is what makes us crack up over that, the truth is, because of Christ, we actually are sisters who are both growing to look more and more like our heavenly Father as time passes.

As long as I've known her, she's been a source of encouragement because not only is she incredibly talented in a bunch of different areas, Carol is a commendable woman for her overall discipline and self-control. After years of my willful rebellious sinful eating when God finally brought me to the point where my eyes were opened to my sin of greed, one of the things He showed me was Carol's life: people wanted to be just like her, even the non-Christians in her life would compare their lives to hers and hope to do better.

All Carol was doing was striving to follow Christ in her life.

It made me think . . . *When the world sees me, whom do I want to look like?* Do I want to look like those in the world whose lives characterized by disorder, discontentment and chaos? Or do I want people who don't follow Jesus to see a growing reflection of my admirable and praiseworthy God? (1 Pet. 2:12).

In the pages of this book, I've written a lot about what God expects. I hope I have done so in a way that helps you see that while He's holy and unrelenting in declaring what is sin, He's actually a very loving and compassionate Father/King. If you've made it to this chapter without skipping, hopefully you have conceded, making the decision to pummel your flesh into submission to God's commands, no matter how much it whines and complains. I know it's really, really hard. I remember how much it ached when I first started to deny my flesh; it wanted to be satisfied! However, let me encourage you again that choosing to obey God in every small thing has great results beyond losing weight.

# Living Love Letters of the Lord to the World at Large

> *"So when they had come together, they were asking Him, saying, "Lord, is it at this time You are restoring the kingdom to Israel?" He said to them, "It is not for you to know times or epochs which the Father has fixed by His own authority; but you will receive power when the Holy Spirit has come upon you; and you shall be My witnesses both in Jerusalem, and in all Judea and Samaria, and even to the remotest part of the earth."* Acts 1:6–8

In your desire to lose this weight, are you looking for a kingdom that can be seen with merely human eyes? Or is your desire to show the world that you serve a King you've yet to see?

I came to the point where I said the words:

"If You can use me . . . " and

"I give it all to You . . . "

Overcoming gluttony alone, or whatever sin you struggle with, isn't the issue. The issue is your surrender to God. Don't make the goal the weight lost, but make the goal of your life to serve God with your obedience. He'll remove the weight when He desires. He wants you to demonstrate *His* work in your life, not *your* work. Yes it does require work on our part, but the reason you do it—the reason I started it—is for the glory of God, and that is how I've persevered all this time and why I get up again every time I fail and regain some weight. Unlike trying to lose weight to get into that dress for your upcoming fancy shindig, there's no deadline to sanctification, just a continual climb toward God.

Once you've surrendered your heart to His rule you have to make a decision to obey. That's all there's to it. A constant string of choices lined up one after another. Just as no one stumbles into sanctification saying, "Oops I'm holy" so no one wakes up one day having become thin overnight. No, you need to choose. However that choice is based on the knowledge that God is better than what you're giving up. Be like Joshua crossing the Jordan when he was commanded to walk into the waters *before they parted,* or like Daniel when he became a vegetarian in the land of the Babylonians so he didn't defile his relationship with God. Be like the apostle Paul in his ministry that led him to proclaim the gospel even though a lot of his successes were rewarded with beatings, hardships, imprisonment, and eventually death, or like Jesus as He faced the cross and the momentary but no less painful separation from His Father, with whom He'd always had a relationship. You need to choose for yourself to obey no matter how hard it is (Josh. 24:15; Dan. 1:8; Phil. 3:13–15; Heb. 12:1–2). The choice isn't whether you'll be thin or not, but is God your precious Lord or not. From there, you'll find the grace and grit to make it through everything, even your own occasional failures.

Don't get me wrong there is nothing wrong with wanting to lose weight, however what is your motivation? If your desire is to please the Lord and not about worldly self-denial and the praise of man, then you'll find you can be patient with the time that it takes to lose the weight as you leave the results up to God. So what are your goals? Is it to make it up a flight of stairs without getting winded? Do you want to run an entire a 5K? Would you like to climb Mount Kilimanjaro? It's all good, if those goals are subordinated to God's will.

It's great to get healthy and all—but it must be for the purpose of serving Him. I find I can accomplish more now that I'm more active (go figure) plus, I'm seeing more opportunities to speak about God to people when they ask me how I've lost the weight and why I do all the things I do. I love how when God truly changes a person's life, He does it in such a way that the person has no choice but to gleefully point back to God as the source of the change. Not a program, nor a food or a drug. Not even a trainer, but God Himself.

I wish I had a magic pill to make it easier—actually no, I don't, because if I had one, then you wouldn't get to learn all the amazing lessons of God and His faithfulness that come as a byproduct of combating your sinful, greedy gluttony. Repenting of any besetting sin is hard, hard work, but the growth comes in the hard work. So while I won't offer you a magic pill, let me at least lead you to the ladder that will take you up toward your goal of daily glorifying God in the area of your killing your sinful appetite.

## Sanctification by Inches, Not Miles

Gaining control of your life as you submit to God in your personal area of struggle is the easiest difficult thing a believer can do. I mean really, look at *any command* in the Bible, matter-of-factually stated; you should be able to just do it, and do so to His glory. However, as we all know, what makes this easy task so difficult is that we don't want to do it.

Yet we still want the external results of an obedient life.

In my case with the weight, all I had to do is not eat as much as I used to and move more than before—except I didn't *want* to do that. Like a little child, I wanted what I wanted and what I wanted was to do whatever I wanted when I wanted—even if it was never. Confusing, huh? Things changed when I decided that what I wanted more was to please God. I had to get control of my Self and make it a slave to God's will, instead of letting it go crazy on its own. I say all this humbly, as I still struggle to run away from things that displease Him.

Of the things I want to control, Self is my least favorite. The times I find it most difficult to control my Self is when I think of the miles I have to go instead of the inches, the years instead of the moments. Concurrent to my bringing my appetite under control, I also tackled the disarray of my home. At one point I told Carol I was slowly succeeding in getting my house clean not by focusing on the whole pig pen I lived in, but only on a square foot of the tabletop at a time. She chirped sweetly, "Inch by inch, it's a cinch. Mile by mile, it's a trial."

It's the same when it comes to subduing your appetite. If I think, *I have to lose seventy-two more pounds (or even thirty pounds) by June,* the task becomes ponderously daunting, but if I think, *I need to eat right and exercise today,* then the task is more manageable. You and I just have to do what I know is right, right now.

In Acts 9:33–35, we read about Peter encountering a man named Aeneas who had been bedridden for eight years due to paralysis. When the apostle healed the man in Jesus' name, Peter gave him this instruction, *"Get up and make your bed."*

He didn't tell this man, "Go out and preach the gospel" (though apparently he must have made the most amazing bed ever, since everyone who lived in his hometown of Lydda gave their lives to the Lord).

Nor did Peter say, "Go into the next room and stretch your legs," or even, "Go out and take a walk down the streets so everyone can see you." No, Peter simply told Aeneas to accomplish the near first thing: "Make your bed." This command was a simple act of self-control so near and accessible that the man couldn't help but do it.

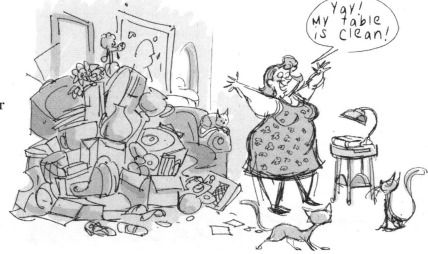

So often when I've been paralyzed by the weight of repenting of my sin, I get even more overwhelmed by the thought that to repent, I must run what amounts to a marathon, starve myself like a prison camp occupant—and will have to live like this FOR

166

THE REST OF MY MISERABLE LIFE!!! I forget that God is glorified by obedient acts in all things, no matter how small (Luke 16:10). Practically speaking, this means that God is just as glorified by my being able to push away from the table when there is more food to be had, as He is if I were to run bravely into a burning building to rescue a child (Mark 12:41-44).

We make pursuit of God much harder than He asks us to. He doesn't ask for wild pledges of great feats—God asks for simple moment-by-moment submission in our tiniest areas.

If you're struggling at being disciplined, take heart. Take smaller bites at your goal, because that's all you have to do. Remember, it's for God's glory. If you're disciplined in the small things He puts right in front of you, you've already had success before the only Audience who really matters. It takes time to get on track or back on track, but it can be done if you do it an inch at a time.

The journey of a thousand miles begins with this step you've already made, if you made the decision to obey God with your appetite. The goals are not the issue, they're candy on the way; God wants you to follow Him.

## Getting Started

Here's what I did when I started. Some of the steps may seem simplistic, but remember a tiny stone, wielded by an unremarkable boy who had faith in an all-powerful God, felled Goliath. Don't take for granted the little things that can produce great results.

*Make a decision to do it*—and then don't have a conversation with yourself afterward...You'll always lose the debate.

*Have a cheering section.* It helps to tell ANYONE WHO'LL LISTEN about your goal of repentance. Then as they see you moving to it they can encourage you and be encouraged as well. (More on this in chapter 14.)

*Go at your own pace.* This isn't a race, it's . . . well I don't know what it is, but it's not a race. I can't stress this point enough. Proverbs 19:2 cautions against being too hasty. It's not just because Solomon hated world records, it's because he recognized people need time to gather tools to function properly, whether it's lessons from God or allowing your body time to adjust to the changes it's undergoing.

God calls us to compare ourselves with ourselves and not others (Gal. 6:4). Yes, there are races and yes, there's only one winner, but in the race to the finish line of life, Christ has already won, so our goal in this race is only to run increasingly better in the footsteps of our big brother, Jesus.

*Make obedience to God's commands your goal, not the weight lost.* Weight comes off in its own slow time. People may not notice, or if they do they may not say anything about it. It shouldn't matter if you're doing it to please the Lord and not man. Though people may or may not give you praise, no one can take away the fact that God was incredibly pleased today because you made that choice. The hardest part of starting is the getting past not wanting to start. There are times when I still find myself thinking, *Ugh, I don't want to do this!* How do I get past it? By remembering I'm doing it for God's glory, and by just focusing on being obedient this moment, right *now*. Obedience is not a one-time thing, but a series of many micro choices. The joy and momentum will eventually come, but for now, you need to exert your determination and force of will to catapult you from the gravitational pull of sinful complacency.

*Expect plateaus.* It's normal for your body to stop losing weight from time to time, but you should know that there are spiritual plateaus as well. There are seasons of drive and determination once you get going, but then, like the skies in a drought, the verve dries up. Poof! In my life, the reasons for this vary from focusing too much on the results, to emotional malaise, or even to other completely non-related events. Sometimes even the great results can cause a plateau as I figure, *I look okay* or *I've been going so hard for a while I can slack off a little.* NO, NO! NO! Danger! Danger! Danger! Again, don't base your success on results (except the results of being more like Christ). Kicking back on the externals will always prove to be a faulty three-legged stool.

Other plateaus may come because your determination vanishes due to emotional heaviness. You're only human; you can't be a spiritual dynamo a hundred percent of the time. In those times of darkness, don't be discouraged if you can't work as hard as you've worked in the past. If you're genuinely not in sin (and even if you are), crawl into the lap of the Lord to find grace in your time of need. It might be that God has pulled the plug on your emotional progress to teach you something in the "land of wait," where your spiritual car's stalled on the side of the road.

While we're at it—*quit checking your progress!* Quit hopping on the scale night and day, every day. The reason not to hop on the scale is obvious: Our bodies aren't always going to do what we want them to do when we want them to do it. So since we're doing this for the glory of God and trusting Him for the results, in His timing, hopping on the scale adds an element of frustration when we don't see the number we were hoping for. So . . . don't do it.

As for the mirror. (Shudder . . . the mirror . . . ) There are consequences to the sin of gluttony: saggy skin, stretch marks, dimples—and I don't mean the cute Cary Grant kind— and we need to accept it as the aftereffects of our rebellion. However beyond those unfortunate remnants of your past infractions, there are other things you see in the mirror as well that aren't true—seeing yourself as ugly, fat, unacceptable; viewing yourself in comparison to what you fantasize about, discounting the fact that you're no longer what you used to be, even long after you've lost a sizable amount of weight. I called it "having fat eyes." For my part, I discovered I wasn't able to see how much weight I lost. I knew I wasn't ginormous, but I also didn't believe it when my friend called me "Skinny McBeanpole."

*Use what you already know of the Bible* (James 1:22). Even without this book, a lot of us are without excuse when it comes to obeying God in appetite submission. We've learned so much about Him in the sermons we hear, the small groups we attend, and even in our personal devotions, that we need to start using what we already know to live in obedience to Him. I heard a story once about POWs during World War II who put together a Bible based on all the verses they collectively knew. It gave them hope even though they didn't have the actual Bible with them. They lived with the scraps of God's word, and it kept them alive. When I first started this journey I thought about the verse in James 4:17 which reads, "Therefore, to one who knows the right thing to do and does not do it, to him it is sin." It made me think, *I wonder how far would I get if I obeyed what I already knew how to do?* (Apparently over a hundred pounds away from where I was five years ago and to other countries and back . . . )

As time went along and the weight slowly began to leave me, I saw how God deals with us in completely individual ways. The food specifics that worked for others hadn't worked for me, but *the principles of obedience* from what I knew from the Bible did. For that, God alone gets the glory.

We always need to keep actively seeking to learn more about God, His ways, and how He wants us to obey Him. But we need to actually be *using* what we already know. A large number of the verses in this book were not looked up to support my points; they were verses I'd already learned through reading my Bible over the years as I sought to grow in Christ. However, I just started using them only five years ago. It's so very sad that it took me so long to pick up God's scriptural bread crumb trail, yet it's encouraging to see that our God has given you and me everything we need to obey Him right now, if we would only use what we've already learned from Him.

**What scriptural tools do you already have in your toolkit to begin approaching the dismantling of your beloved sin? Take some time today and write them down—even if you can think of only one. Pray and ask God to help you apply that to your life.**

This will work if you are not a believer, as well. If you've made it this far in the book you already know enough to radically turn your life on its ear. You now know the gospel. You

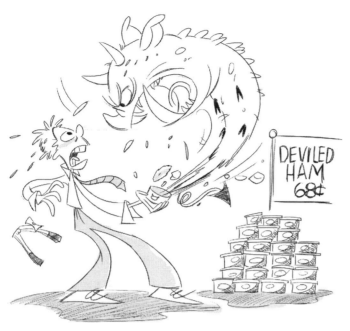

know the benefits of a life to come as opposed to the destruction waiting for you. Above all, you know how much God loves you in the midst of this broken old world. Your first act of obedience to what you know should be to come to Him for forgiveness and salvation.

In this sense, there's no difference between a Christian and a non-Christian—we all have to make a choice to do what we already know. We all have to put on our big kid pants one leg at a time to see eventual results.

*There's no bad food.* I know, shocking. More on this in chapter 12, *"Don't Hate What You Ate."* The problem, as I hope you understand by now, is not what we eat, but rather how much we eat. Of course I understand there are food allergies; some foods that will quite literally kill some people if eaten, but that's not everyone's issue. Most of us just eat too much of a good thing.

*Think before you eat.* I don't know about you, but I pretty much scarf my food down without giving it much thought. Then approximately two bites before the end of whatever I'm eating I think, *Oh dear, that was really good . . .* Then the dissatisfaction with not having any more of it descends on me like a cloud. We need to slooooow down. Actually take a moment to think about what you're eating when you're eating it. I learned to do this by applying 2 Corinthians 10:3–5:

> *For though we walk in the flesh, we do not war according to the flesh, for the weapons of our warfare are not of the flesh, but divinely powerful for the destruction of fortresses. We are destroying speculations and every lofty thing raised up against the knowledge of God, **and we are taking every thought captive to the obedience of Christ.*** (emphasis mine)

The Bible commands us to take every thought captive, but us of the greedy bent really don't think about what we're shoveling in our mouths. Seriously . . . would you be such a little gobbler if you truly thought about how much you were eating and how you looked while doing it? Consider the simple mundane task of eating as an opportunity to slow your pace and let your thoughts circle back so that they can be caught. The extra time you devote to eat more slowly may make the difference between finding victory or thinking, *Well I blew it by eating too much, so I might as well douse myself with gasoline and set myself on fire!* Slow down. Enjoy your food. Think about what a gift God's given you on your plate in front of you.

*Be grateful for what you eat.* The other side of thinking about what you ate is being thankful for it. Seriously, do you even think about what you eat or do you just shovel it into your mouth? We worship the taste and texture of food, and oftentimes something that's meant to power the machine gets converted into a hobby and a pacifier. It was never designed to be those things. Sport eating is like people who hop indiscriminately in and out of the sack because it feels good. Just as the pleasure in sex was designed to bond a husband and wife together and make creating life a joy and not a chore, so the pleasure of eating comes through its great tastes, so it's not a strain to get it down. We should be thankful; truly thankful to God we get food that suits our tastes, not to mention the fact that He provides us our food in the first place. (Again, more on this in chapter 12.)

*Trust God for the results* (Ps. 37:3–6). Are you cultivating faithfulness? Are you being firm in your land? Not faithful for the results, but steadfast for the sake of growing in whatever area God has called you to submit to Him in obedience. Sometimes our lands are green and flowing with everything we think will make us happy; other times its pretty dry and desert-y . . . kind of like my back yard because of our California drought. God adjures us to show fidelity wherever we find ourselves. Good or bad, fair or foul. "Be faithful," He says.

Be faithful for its very own sake, and not because of any reward. It's plenty easy to be faithful when you're competing for a $250,000 prize, but is that faithfulness, really? I know for me, focusing on the reward makes me surly when I don't get it when I think I should. "Uh, I've been working long at this faithfulness thing. Isn't it about time You should make good on your end of the bargain? Hello, God, can you hear me? Hello?" I'm just being honest, and then I confess that to God and seek to change my focus. Be stalwart for the sake of obeying Him, and not because of some perceived carrot dangling out there in the distance.

Would you be steadfast even when no one is there to reward you? Would you make your bed and keep your house neat if you were single? Would still you go work out even if you scale didn't budge a pound for weeks? (Or worse, went up?) Yes, God does promise to give us the desires of our hearts—but His timing is not our own. That desire might not be fulfilled until the distant future . . . or even maybe after we die and see Him. Will you cultivate faithfulness anyway?

*Change your attitude toward repentance.* Repentance is an ongoing act. Not just the coming to the cross the first time and saying, "God forgive me." For every time we read something in the Bible with which we disagree we have to see that it is a battle of wills at that point, and in this staring contest, God is the one who won't blink. We eventually will obey, because well, God always wins, but rather than seeing those occurrences as God looking down on us like the grumpy cat, saying, "Repent because I told you so," look at it this way: He says "Repent, for I LOVE you so." We need to see God's commands as directions given in love.

View each act of obedient eating not as a draught of poison, but an antidote to save you (Rom. 2:4). It may not feel like it at times, but each time we choose to obey God in repentance, we're actually being healed while our flesh is being killed.

*View your trials as trainers, not tormentors.* Use each setback in circumstances to seek God and His will in your life. Let your trials help you grow instead of using them as excuses to eat (James 1:2–3). Most people identify negative emotions as their most common reason for eating when they're not hungry. Over the past several years I've come to see the deeper reason for my eating; it's more than being sad, bored, angry or lonely; it's just I want to pamper my flesh. That's not to say your feelings don't matter, but address the feelings, not the flesh. If you're bored, go find something to do, whether it's with someone or *for* someone; boredom is a choice, not a destination. If you're sad, you should be praying, appealing to God on the basis of His loving character. Once you've prayed about your sadness, trust Him to take care of it and then think about hopeful things, *not* the issues that brought you despair (Phil. 4:4–8).

I don't want to make light of depression. It's palpable, like a wall or a mountain; the negative emotions are so big they take on a form of their own. For years I wasn't depressed, but I had a low-grade anger going on. It wasn't anger at anyone; it was just there, like emotional B.O. I found the key to take care of it: letting go of my beloved sin. Sin blocks our communication with God. He doesn't leave us, because He's committed to us. But when we sin, it stops up our ears to hearing God, who is the source of truth.[17] The temptation when you're sad is to pull into yourself and go it alone, but not only is that selfishness, it's like shooting yourself in the foot to cease listening to God's limitless wisdom and relying on your limited smarts (Prov. 18:1).

If you've prayed to come to the point of really forsaking your beloved sin, whether its greed or something else God has revealed to you along the way, and you're still languishing, reach out to a friend or reach out to the body of Christ. Sometimes it helps to find hope with some skin on, sometimes you just need a hug. But those aren't the first things you should

---

[17] For those who fall prey to emotional eating regarding sadness, go back and check out the Scriptures below; come to God for truth instead of blocking His truth by turning to food. The psalmist was in real despair. But when he poured out his heart to the Lord, he was able to find Him trustworthy. By holding on to sin we dam our spiritual ears from hearing truth and thus miss out on the very thing that can help us in our trial. Use the key of forsaking your pet sins to find release from your prison of despair. Scriptures about turning to God for truth—Ex. 34:6; Ps. 25:4–5, 10; 31:5; 40:10; 43:3–4; 57:2–3, 10; 69:13; 71:22; 86:15; 111:7–8; John 14:6.

run to, otherwise they become just like food, something else to take the place of God.

*No repentance pity parties.* Losing weight by being obedient takes hard, hard work (Phil. 2:12–16). I've lost track of the times I've heard people blame their inability to overcome their besetting sin on their lack of faith. It's not a lack of faith that keeps us mired in stagnation—it's our lack of work. God has given us everything we need to accomplish His will. For one, He's revealed His will to us in the Bible. Two, He's given us the power through regeneration to accomplish His will. The only thing that's missing from the equation is our elbow grease.

It's as if a master chef gave us his secret recipe, bought us the ingredients, set us in his kitchen and said, "Go forth and bake a cake." What more do you need? Bake. The. Cake. It isn't always easy to do. Sometimes you drop eggshells in the batter or you get distracted and forget to add the vanilla or even leave the cake in the oven so it burns, then you start over. However if you follow the master chef's recipe you're going to make a cake, even if you make a mess while doing it. It's the same with obeying God's commands. Quit waiting to feel like doing it. That's not part of the equation: *"commands + X = sanctification"*. The X is your hard work.

*Remember the end isn't really the end.* I don't say this to be discouraging, but realistically, when have you found true and lasting satisfaction in achieving that long-sought-after prize? Goals are fine, but in the end we need to hold the achievement of them loosely because who knows when or if you'll reach them (James 4:13–16). Tons of people lose scads of weight in a flash. Remember, God wants to change the hidden person of your heart. Am I giving myself an out for being five years into this process and still having twenty pounds left to lose? I don't think so. You see, I continue to learn and grow in the process of losing and gaining and losing a bit more . . . and gaining some back. *UGH* Yet, I will never be 312 pounds

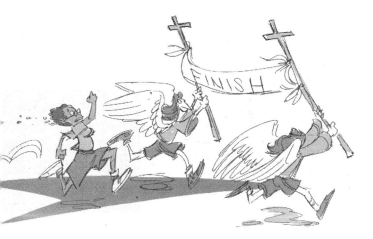

*Hebrews 12:1-3*

again, I know too much of God's faithfulness and His commands to return to that sin like a dog to vomit.

So while I'm not done and I keep working to get to my goal, God still digs away at my heart using my desire to lose this weight as the doorway to point out all kinds of other hideous things I didn't realize were lurking in my character.

So these are the practical attitudes I adopted to lose this weight. In the end, what has enabled me to endure is the greater goal of seeking to know God better and become more like Him. I don't know what my future holds. I might make it just five pounds short of my goal and be struck by a meteor—hey it could happen . . .

Okay, how about a lightning bolt?

Will I be a failure for not having achieved my goal? No. God has bought my victory with the shed blood of Jesus. His goal was to cut the sin of fat from my heart, and while getting the blubber off my butt is important to me—I always want to remember what God thinks is most important: to have a lean heart spiritually.

## Brain Surgeons, Not Bums

Someone once wrote on Facebook: "Hard to get back into the routines of life."

To which I quipped jokingly . . . "I suppose it depends on which routines you mean. I mean it would be more difficult to get back to being a brain surgeon than being a hobo."

Immediately my joke made me think. The fact that life is challenging is actually a blessing. The blessing is that our challenges reveal our true identity. The reason things are difficult to do at times may just be because of who we are. It's more challenging to slip into the routines of the son or daughter of a King than those of a lowly commoner!

We need to rejoice for the tough routines that God calls us to live in, because it means we've been transferred from the kingdom of darkness into the kingdom of light. From bum to brain surgeon. If you are a Christian, I encourage you to remember just who you are today and why you live (Eph. 4:15).

Both trials and blessings have been my tests. God uses them to determine the soundness of the work He is doing in me and then He points me to the cures to heal the weaknesses the trials and blessings have revealed. If I looked at my individual failures to stay on my diet as only fleshly missteps instead of spiritual revelations, eventually I could chose to stop working, because as we get older, who really cares what we look like, right? Isn't all this focus on appearance merely a thing of vanity for the young?

No. Never forget our actions have more than a fleshly consequence. Though we'll never feel the eternal sting of the fires of hell, God uses our trials and blessings to burn off the attitudes that won't be fit for heavenly living.

God doesn't save sinners and grant them the wisdom to repent and the power to do so in order that they may be a super race of humans that walk this earth. No, quite the opposite; God shows us all our failings and then gives us the power to overcome them to show us how indescribably needy we are. I now have the power to get up every time I fail, but the point is; *I fail.* I'm not eternally strong and powerfully focused. Perfection isn't mine, nor will it ever be this side of heaven. I don't just need God to help me walk through the day. I don't just need God to forgive me when I fail. *I. Need. God.* Knowing God doesn't weaken me, but knowing God reveals my weakness.

So we persevere because of this: Christians have the privilege of being called His children. God knows our names, and He is intimately acquainted with all that's going on with us. This means that His actions toward us, no matter how taxing they may feel to us, are filtered through His attributes of grace, justice, mercy, holiness, and love.

So many of the problems we face are caused by something deeper than their external manifestations. God's transformation does produce external results. You'll lose weight, or successfully make your way past a host bar at a lavish wedding if you're someone who struggles with drunkenness, or turn down the advance by the hot unsaved guy if your temptation is lust. Focus on addressing the sinful matters of your selfish heart as He reveals them and you'll get the results thrown in. If you focus merely on the externals, you'll eventually lose them no matter how hard you've worked to gain them.

# Life After the Fireworks

If we're only doing it for the goal of having gotten it done, we'll find the satisfaction in the end hollow and seek something else to fill that hollowness that only God alone should fill. This does not apply only to seeking jobs, relationships or anything else as a goal for satisfaction; losing weight for the sake of losing weight alone can be just as empty. We people can put a lot of work into achieving things like weight loss that in the end prove to be meaningless.

There's a town in Iowa. It's so small that the water tower bearing its name is almost as big as the town square. My friend Beth has relatives who live there. One time during the winter many years ago, she and I went for a visit and I noticed among other things—besides the vast corn fields in some places and the pervasive smell of hogs in others—several collection receptacles for aluminum cans simply labeled "Fireworks." The town is so small they can't afford public fireworks, so they work all year, saving cans for recycling, doing dances, raffles and whatever else they can think of to raise money to have a special day on July 4. That touched me. I wanted to live in a town so patriotic that they would work hard all year to have their fourth of July be perfect.

So I impressed on my friend I wanted to return and experience a real Midwestern 4th of July, and we did. It was a wonderful time with her family. We had a milk-can supper,[18] set off fireworks of our own and even had a momentary scare that the community fireworks might be called off because of rain. Eventually, though, the clouds parted, and the town came out for the parade, the cow chip bingo, then some more rain and finally everyone hunkered

---

[18]  A milk-can supper is a stew of meat and vegetables cooked on an open flame in a can that is used to collect the milk from the cow, which looks sort of like a giant teakettle.

down as the dusk turned into inky night. I brought my video camera to document the whole thing. I was so excited to see their excitement for all their hard work and effort.

As the first popping blooms of fireworks went off in the sky, I was impressed because it was quite a show. I hopped to my feet with my camera and ran along the front of the crowd to get reaction shots . . . However, as I looked at their faces I was surprised to see, not childlike delight and awe, or even joy, but an impassive and flaccid boredom. In the end many of them looked away and said, "Okay, this part is done with, where can we get a beer?"

Sure it wasn't everyone . . . but I was intrigued by the level of underwhelm I saw that night.

Weight loss goals can be like that . . . Don't get me wrong—goals are great! But if all you have is weight loss as your goal it's kind of like an ellipses rather than a period at the end of a sentence. Then what? We need to realize the things we achieve in life are just temporary. Of course that doesn't mean we don't strive to hit them, but we need to reframe our expectations for them. There's something exciting about the anticipation of a hoped-for dream but when we get there, we see the result as a little hollow and seek for something else that maybe might be a little better. . . After all the work, we see the vanity in the end. Our worldly goals can prove to be empty if there's not a heavenly motivation for them.

In heaven we won't have weight issues, because there we'll be self-controlled. We'll also be patient, loving, gentle, kind, and considerate of others. We need to combine our goals. For example: "I want to be the kindest size six ever!" or "I want to patiently put my sister in Christ first and run with her every once in a while, even though I really don't like talking while I'm exercising." You'll find that seeking to achieve the goal of "less weight" becomes more satisfying if your main goal is growing in Christlikeness.

This is a lifetime character change we need to remember. Not just making it to the finish line and then wandering around with a "Well, now what? Where do I go to get that beer?" look on our face. That kind of attitude shows that we have forgotten why we began in the first place: to live on earth now by the rules God has for us in heaven.

We need to remind ourselves constantly of our true goal. It isn't so we can get a whole new wardrobe, improve our relationships, perk up our health or get a promotion at work. The goal of our faithfulness should always be to hear our Father say: *"Well done, good and faithful slave. You were faithful with a few things, I will put you in charge of many things; enter into the joy of your master"* (Matt. 25:23).

The goal is to hear our Father when we join Him in the kingdom of heaven.

## Meanwhile—Here on Earth

Therefore regarding the time it takes to lose your weight, I hope this relieves the weight on your shoulders about your . . . well, your weight. God has saved you no matter what the condition of your body. He does, however, care about your obedience. It's good to have your weight be at a healthy level because it helps you serve Him and others better, it gives you more energy, and prevents people from judging you about your apparent lack of self-control. BUT, if the weight doesn't melt away immediately, or you don't get big muscles fast, or gain the ability to run a marathon by tomorrow—don't beat yourself up over your gradual physical progress. Instead, take encouragement that your focus on the hidden character of your heart is right in line with God's will for you as His child.

As you're faithful and God wills, in time the weight will come down, your heart will become stronger, your lungs will process air better, your muscles will look better, you will move more deftly, etc. Develop faithfulness to obedience from the heart to seek the rule of Kingdom of God in your heart by doing that which He's given you in each moment as it unfolds before you. Jesus Himself encouraged His disciples that even the tiniest amount of faith could have a great result (Mark 4:30–32).

That's why in the end I remind myself to take lightly what I see in the mirror. My tape measure can only measure what can be seen, and my scale will only give me a false sense of accomplishment—or a frustrating sense of lack of one. I prefer to remember to see myself through God's eyes, to measure myself by His Word, and to weigh my actions by His standards.

If understanding the basics of God is like building a house before you paint it, then what we've just discussed is like putting on the primer. You need to have these attitudes in place so everything else you seek to paint into your life in obedience to God will actually stick. All of these attitudes can be summed up in a few words: obey God and be patient, as you trust Him for the results. Now we'll go into the next chapters and put on the various colors of paint in the areas of eating, exercise, knowing where to go for help, and being a help to others.

> *Feed me with the food that is my portion,*
> *That I not be full and deny You and say, "Who is the Lord?"*
> *Or that I not be in want and steal,*
> *And profane the name of my God.*
> — *Prov. 30:8b–9*

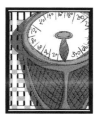

# Take A-Weigh

- God's commands are not as complicated as we make them.
- Live your life in obedience to Him as a testimony to the world.
- Having a growing relationship with God should be our goal, otherwise our results will prove to be meaningless.

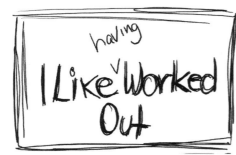

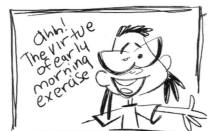

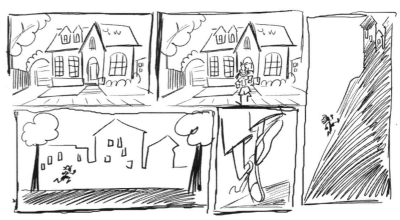

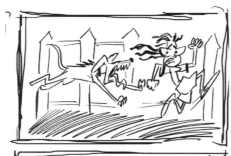

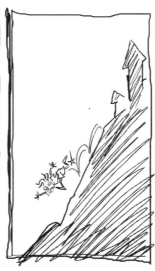

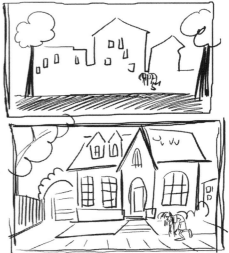

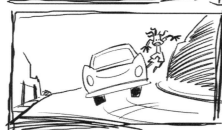

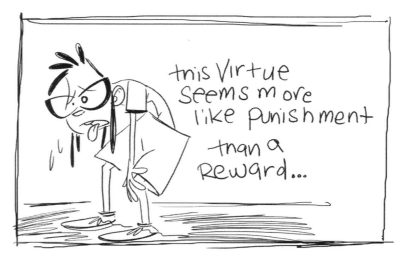

Chapter 11

# Going to the Bank

> *Do you not know that those who run in a race all run, but only one receives the prize? Run in such a way that you may win. Everyone who competes in the games exercises self-control in all things. They then do it to receive a perishable wreath, but we an imperishable. Therefore I run in such a way, as not without aim; I box in such a way, as not beating the air; but I discipline my body and make it my slave, so that, after I have preached to others, I myself will not be disqualified.*     *1 Cor. 9:24–26*

It was your garden-variety, large-sized pickup truck, the kind you would see at a construction site. What made me nervous was the man behind its wheel. I was out jogging my normal route and even though I wasn't wearing my glasses, I could see the truck and its driver about half a block away. He was just sitting there . . . engine idling . . . staring at me. *At least I thought he was . . .* I couldn't be sure . . . but maybe? Oh . . . golly . . . I dunno.

So slowly I jogged to the other side of the street (for that's the only speed I had, slow). I wasn't going to be the victim of some creepy freak in a garden-variety construction site pickup truck! However as I neared the idling vehicle, the man behind the wheel shouted out in a thick Middle Eastern accent, "Are you a loser?"

I wrinkled my eyes and squinted at him. As I said, I couldn't see, and not being able to see made it somewhat difficult to hear as well.

"Huh?"

I answered back with suspicion but kept my distance: I'd seen this slide show when I was in elementary school. *He wasn't going to snatch me off the street!*

"Are you a LOSER?" he repeated, this time a bit louder, with an affable air.

Then it dawned on me that this absolute stranger was encouraging me. His reference to losers was the extreme body makeover series where several morbidly obese people lock themselves away on a ranch where dieticians coach and personal trainers yell at them for ten months with the hope that they will not only lose weight, but be the one remaining person who wins a cash cow of twenty-five thousand dollars!

"Uh . . . yeah?"

"Keep it up!!" He said, adding a friendly thumbs-up for encouragement.

By that point I'd lost over a hundred and twenty pounds with the goal of losing the last forty-two, and strangers like this man had been encouraging me all the way all along my journey, from the little boy who called me fat when I first started, to a woman more recently, out with her walking partner, who said, "You're skinny!" as she passed me going the other way. Everyone felt they needed to weigh in on my workout and weight loss. Each time they did, it brought a smile to my face and I thanked God for His providential gift of this random group of cheerleaders. Though I wasn't working out to be noticed there was something encouraging in seeing that I wasn't alone.

## Depleting Our Bank Accounts

One of the more difficult aspects of losing weight is actually coming up with ways to help it go. While I still believe that a continuous pattern of eating too much causes us to store fat and eating less food gives you an opportunity to use some of it, I also believe there is another way to help move some of that fat out of storage and that way is—gasp—*exercising*.

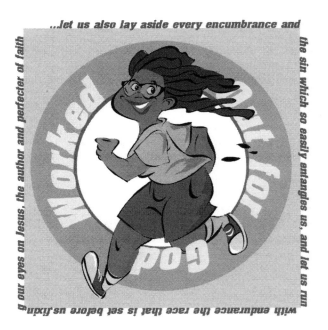

DUN-DUN-DAHHHHH!

No, duh. We all know this, so why have I put this chapter in a book that's largely a spiritual primer on dealing with the sin that puts on long-term weight? The reason is that so many people in the church *don't do it because they hate it*. They treat exercise as a preference rather than a prescription for life, which it is, and try as I might, I'll never find a verse that says, "Thou Shalt Spend Twenty Minutes in the Gym Three to Five Days a Week or Else You're Not Saved." But that doesn't mean we can't find something beneficial in it. Everyone knows about the health benefits of a consistent course of committed physical activity, but there can be transforming spiritual benefits, as well.

When I first started, I wasn't a big fan of exercising myself and had to find ways to motivate myself to do it (even if that motivation was to say that I liked *having done it*). I confess that even to this day I go in and out of wanting to do it, but when I'm faithful to get out there in the end, I'm always happy that I did it. Exercising consistently is a proven method of helping take care of the evidences of our overindulgences.

Remember, the body is actually doing its job super-well when we get fat. It's just storing up resources for when there's a famine . . . *Cha—as if!* Of course, instead of storing for a famine, we've become a people who practice being food misers in our greed.

Every time you put something in your mouth, you're essentially covenanting with your body that you're going to use it rather than store it. It's as if you said, "I just ate 3472 calories worth of pizza because I'm going to spend half the day chain-sawing a forest of trees." When we break that contract and don't cut down those trees—or even walk around the block for that matter—we gain weight through fat storage. Then the temptation is to panic and to try to throw everything off the ship in a sense, by starving ourselves. However, what happens is we don't only throw away the bad stuff, we also throw away some of the good.

Starving yourself is known to deteriorate your muscles, hurt your heart, weaken your immune system, deplete vital nutrients in your body, cause temporary dehydration, and slow down your metabolism—which means you'll need *fewer* calories to make fat. Yikes! Not to mention that food deprivation affects your mood so it makes you *gwumpy!* But it's a fast fix, so everybody does it.

We live in a time of instant gratification; our money seems to burn a hole in our pockets and we can't wait to spend it. But the fat we've saved? Not so much. Now when confronted with the idea that your hoarding is sin, the temptation is to starve yourself to deal with the consequences, but our loving Father has given us a more gentle way to deal with the consequences of our sin; a way that builds patience, discipline, faithfulness and gratitude. God has given us a way to spend the fat we've stored in a way that will actually build our bodies while depleting our dietary stores. In His kindness He has provided a means to lose the weight that doesn't involve torture (well, at least not the kind you'd find in medieval times) and even builds in the carrot of endorphins, the feel-good hormone that your body produces when you exercise.

We can repent of taking in food and not using it by purposely exercising beyond the level of activity we would do in a normal day. This is something like the idea of letting your yes be yes and your no be no (James 5:12). When you overeat, it's as if your appetite has said, *Yes I intend on doing something spectacular with this enormous amount of food I'm about to consume*—when all the time it's lying. But when we exercise, we can be like little Zaccheus, who not only stopped defrauding people, but after giving half his possessions to the poor, he paid back fourfold anyone he had cheated (Luke 9:1-10). He did more than just stop doing wrong; he went the extra mile and gave more. We too can do the same when we do more than just eating less.

While the commitment to exercise may not be giving to the poor, it does stop you from

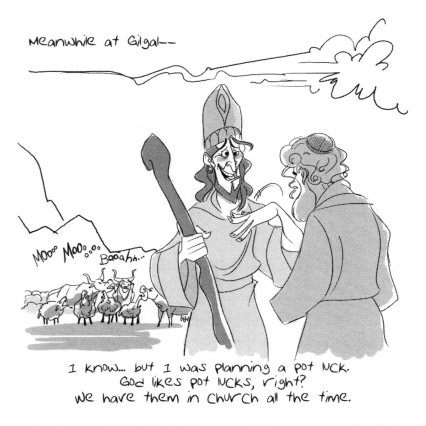

Meanwhile at Gilgal—

Mooo Moo.... Baaahh...

I know... but I was planning a pot luck. God likes pot lucks, right? We have them in church all the time.

stealing from others.

When you're not physically at your best, you rob people of the service you could be to them. You steal from your husband because you're too tired to clean the house or make love. You defraud your children because you lack the energy to play with them. You rob God when you're so physically unsure of yourself that you won't go on a mission trip because you're afraid you won't be able to do what's required in another land.

Now that we know our fat store represents sinful hoarding, we need to deplete it, but rather than just pulling the plug on the bathtub of our greed, let's get out a bucket and bail! Spend what you've saved!

Spend it on baseball; spend it on runs! Spend it on swimming or anything physically fun. Spend it on skating or the flying trapeze: set aside time to do what you please. Just spend it! I found my reason for recommending exercise in addition to moderate eating rather than starving ourselves in 1 Samuel 15:22 where king Saul was rebuked for not doing what the Lord told him to do. He figured he would disobey God and give up something later. God wasn't down with that idea and He told him that he wanted obedience, not sacrifice. In this case, it's actually obedience to work out, because you're using the food for its intended purpose.

## This Useful Old Grass

I had a friend who used to joke and say the Proverbs 31 woman (Prov. 31:17) worked out and had great arms. But the Bible warns that those who are physically strong alone do not have everything they need (Pss. 33:16; 90:10; 147:10–11). You and I need only look at the example of Samson's life to see that being physically strong gets a person into big trouble if they're not devoted to the Lord (Judg. 13:24–16:31).

Our bodies are like the grass: We start young and strong, but because of sin, disease and gravity, we get weak, decrepit and eventually die. We have the encouragement through the Bible that our bodies aren't necessarily the bodies we'll have in eternity.

And yet . . .

The apostle Paul in 1 Timothy 4:8 wrote to the young pastor, *"bodily discipline is only of little profit . . . "* But he didn't say, *"no profit."*

The world in its view of physical fitness is wrong-minded in their approach. They seek to stave off death while killing themselves with relentless physical activity. However, we in the church are just as guilty of having a wrong view of working out; by not doing it we kill our effectiveness for God. How can we hope to accomplish the things He has planned specifically for us if our inactivity means we can't even make it up a flight of stairs without huffing and puffing?

Yes: God made you and I for specific purposes, but are you hamstringing yourself because you're too lazy to do a few leg-lifts?

The days of our lives were written down before there was yet one of them (Ps. 139:16). God won't take our lives a moment before our pre-ordained time, nor will He let us overstay. . . But we can affect the quality of our lives as we circle the sun on this ball of dirt year after year.

A person who exercises consistently, even moderately, has more energy and can do more things than a person who doesn't. It's not about looking hot in your new slinky red dress. It's just simple mathematics. Activity begets the power to be active as your muscles make you more graceful. Training your respiratory system gives you more oxygen to sustain the demands of your more active body.

However most people don't work out because it's too painful to do it. If they do make it out the door, the thought they have to do it day after day after day after day becomes too daunting for them, so they just give up. I remember how hard it was to walk when I was so circus huge; it was difficult for me to drag my elephantine mass around the block: I hated it.

## Getting Over the Hurdle of Trying to Get Over the Hurdles

So what got me going when I was in so much knee pain going uphill that I had to walk up the incline sideways? What made me keep going when every bit of my being was like *Please, kill me now!!!* In my embarrassment I lumbered past an old Armenian man who had no English but could still applaud and give me the thumbs up approval: *Yes, giant woman, I see your good deeds and I urge you on!*

I'd read somewhere it takes twenty-one days to make a habit, so I thought, "Okay, I'll give this thing twenty one days and hopefully by then my brain will be into it . . . "

Every day I'd drag myself out of bed, put on my fancy new kicks, raggedy shorts and stained T-shirt and think as I plodded down the street, "This is day one (or day two or day three) . . . of twenty-one" Every day, I'd do the math in my head and take comfort in myself that *this day* was one day closer to twenty one where the habit will be set and I'm one day father away from one where I didn't want to do anything. Eventually, I stopped doing the

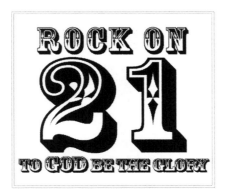

math—I guess that's when the habit began to firm up. So I started another round of twenty ones with a different route to set it, counting until I no longer needed to do so.

Sometimes when I lose my motivation, I have to go back to that point and restart my 21s. It's my way of reminding myself I need to focus on today when I've become overwhelmed with the relentlessness of doing the hard task of maintaining the discipline of exercise every day UNTIL I DIE!!!!

I've learned two things from this process of learning to navigate those relentless mundane tasks. The first is found in the words of Jesus' Sermon on the Mount, where He told His listeners to not worry about tomorrow because today had enough worries of its own (Matt. 6:34). The application to exercising is this: It's hard, some days more difficult than others. There are days when I feel I'm the fastest and strongest woman on the planet, but there are other days when I feel like I'm dragging the weight of the planet behind me. Those incredibly painful, sluggish days are enough to not only wipe out the times when I felt as though I was Wonder Woman, but they also have the power to send me whimpering back to the comfort of my house and computer chair. But understand this, those sluggish days have that kind of power only because I project them into the future.

In a sense, I not only drag the real weight of the world today, but I add to it, the *supposed* weight of the world I'll have to drag tomorrow. It makes today's agony much worse than it actually is. While I'm working out today, the mere thought of the relentlessness of difficulty as the weeks go by is enough to make me feel more tired than I would be if I just ran with only *that day's* run in mind. Jesus' reminder to think only on today lightens the load. We don't know what's going to happen tomorrow. It might be just as bad as today. . . It could be worse . . . OR—*it could be better.*

We only have to exercise today. We don't have to work out today for *tomorrow.* Why make it harder on ourselves than we need to? To be honest, we could be dead tomorrow, for all we know. So exercise today and repent today, do all today as you seek to have God's kingdom come in your life.

# Finding the Hidden Treasure in the Humdrum Workout

The other thing I learned in the process of working out each day was that doing it produced the by-product of faithfulness.

As I made my way through the slow and arduous progress of daily movement, I was encouraged not by the results alone, but also by the growth of character as I learned to be faithful to just keep doing it despite the results. While it's a stretch to find commands to go out and exercise, God *does tell us to cultivate faithfulness* (Ps. 37:3). You would think the command to cultivate faithfulness would be equivalent to planting it as a little baby seed and watching it grow, but that's not the case. Actually the word for cultivate in the Hebrew means to shepherd or be a friend of. It's almost the idea that faithfulness is there for us, but we need to care for it, and grow a relationship with it.

Think of the friends you've had for a long time who can finish your sentences and laugh at the same stupid inside jokes. That didn't happen when you first met one another. You were awkward and clunky. You had a connection, something that made you want to keep coming back to know more about this person, but you were going to have to keep at it to crack that nut. God's command to cultivate faithfulness is pretty much the same way. Faithfulness is the best friend you'll ever have, because with it, you will be able to accomplish all God calls you to tackle, from dealing with the sin within your heart to sharing the gospel with people even when they say "no." Faithfulness is being trustworthy. Your friend faithfulness will be there by your side to egg you on, *if you cultivate it, even when it concerns small matters.*

Faithfulness is an important aspect of shepherding, a task that involves repetition, with little thanks or fanfare. Look at the life of a shepherd. Herd animals were the life of early Old Testament peoples, providing both their food and clothing. They indicated how wealthy or poor their owners were, which made it an all-important job to care for them. There wasn't a lot of excitement in tending a herd of sheep and goats, which really is a good thing, because a flock, like money the in the bank, should be allowed to grow at a consistent rate without a lot of surprises. A shepherd's job was pretty much the same day after day. He'd get up, take the sheep for a stroll to find them food and water while it was still cool and then take them someplace during the heat of the day to hang out in the shade. After that, he'd take them someplace else to feed and water them again and at last take them home. It wasn't a very exciting or demanding job but the shepherd had to be faithful. The flock of a shepherd who wasn't faithful to the routine would eventually dwindle. No flock meant no livelihood and no life.

Viewing the task of exercise as an important daily event that builds more than physical stamina can elevate our acceptance of doing it. We mistakenly think we could be more productive doing something else that's less like work because it's less boring. Yet being faithful

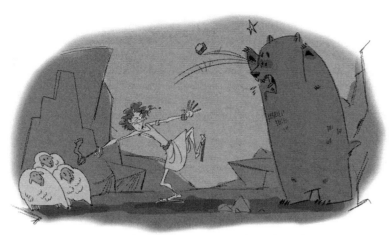

*Before there are giants there will doubtless be bears.*

in this seemingly humdrum yet incredibly important thing means being enriched in other areas.

The world recognizes the importance of faithfulness. Recently I read that job recruiters look favorably on people who run marathons or climb mountains, not because they run marathons or climb mountains, but because of the day-to-day faithfulness involved in training for those giant achievements. A lot of us in the church get discouraged by our insignificant positions in life, while quite often we're the hold-up to our own progress. God saves the weak, and gets the glory for their success, but He also calls those who are weak to be faithful with the tasks He puts before them. If you don't have a big fancy position in your life right now, if you're not married and you want to be, if you're not fulfilling some ministry and you want to do so, maybe it's because God is giving you the opportunity to cultivate faithfulness in the areas you're lax in. If you're not lazy and you do those little things faithfully, irksome as they are, you'll see your responsibilities grow like a shepherd's flock.

Looking at faithfulness in the life of David before he was the King of Israel, we see that as a shepherd boy he endured long, hot days with nothing more than a herd of sheep for company, which gave him plenty of time to sing and write poetry, but really nothing super-challenging—*for the most part*. However, when the Philistines came to attack Israel and David found himself delivering lunch to his older brothers, the youth's faithfulness (and faith that the seemingly untenable situation could be resolved victoriously) was rewarded.

David's skeptical brother reminded him that he was not only a mere shepherd, but also a shepherd *with a little flock* (1 Sam. 17). Yet David was undaunted, for he could see what the king and his army failed to see; the teenager saw God's hand that had power to deliver His people, because he'd seen God's deliverance during his days of being a shepherd of his little flock (1 Sam 17:34–37). Not only did David kill Goliath, but he later cultivated faithfulness to God's call as he fled from King Saul. Finally he himself became king of Israel. Though he'd been tapped to be a king as a boy, God had to equip him for the task of ruling Israel by giving him numerous small ways to cultivate faithfulness.

Jesus gives examples of the progression of someone who's faithful in little things, followed by bigger ones (Matt. 25:14–29). In the parable of the talents, the master calls each of the servants to be faithful to their ability, and then when he sees their results, the master rewards them with more responsibilities in which to be faithful. It was only the servant who wasn't faithful in what he was given (for whatever reason he'd cooked up in his head), who was told that he was lazy and wicked (Matt. 25:26).

Ouch.

If you search your heart, that's the bottom line. We don't like to do things that require work—like working out. Things that may be uncomfortable, that may force us to put in effort and that require consistent faithfulness challenge our willpower. Frankly, I'm with you . . . ughghhghghgh. I'd rather just pull the covers back over my head.

In this task of spending what we've hoarded, we need to press on in the mundane activities that we have decided to do; if we don't we're just being lazy. Take encouragement in this that God isn't being a bully when He asks us to be faithful. He has greater plans than what we can see right in front of us and He promises us a rainbow at the end of our storms (Gal. 6:9).

# Faithful for That Which You Can't See—Yet

Cultivating faithfulness is not all liver and spinach with a castor oil chaser. There's an Easter egg for those who're faithful with the mundane: the reward is that God will give them the desires of their heart (Ps. 37:4).

*Yeah, baby! I'mma be faithful so God will give me that hot new—*

Hooold on a second there. That's not what I'm saying at all!

While God does command us to prayerfully come to Him with our needs and desires, He is only obligated to answer those prayers in accordance with His will and plan (1 John 5:14). Sometimes the best answer to those prayers is yes, sometimes no, and sometimes wait. Let me address the wait.

Remember when I talked about finding the tools in the land of wait? Sometimes, unbeknownst to us, a desire we long for is heavy, large and unwieldy, at least for someone who hasn't built up the muscles of character to handle the fulfillment of that desire. We can ask God for bigger tasks or greater purposes, but maybe He waits to respond because we haven't the strength to accomplish what we asked for. If we insist on not being faithful in the areas of our life we find insignificant, we'll miss the chance to grow in character. More importantly, we'll fail to learn of God's trustworthiness to come to our aid when we're faced with our weakness. Remember that in the long run God knows the greatest gift He can give us is a relationship with Him. He knows that if He granted us our desires immediately, we'd crumble under the pressure when faced with some even more daunting challenge, and we certainly wouldn't turn to Him.

I have found that the concept of cultivating faithfulness in exercising applies to many areas of my life. I know it seems pretty obvious to some, but it wasn't to me. It's not just exercise that falls through the cracks when we walk away from doing right what's in front of us. If we're slack and faithless in one area of our lives, we'll more than likely be slack in others. Cultivating faithfulness is a constant choice.

I know lots of us are short on time to exercise, but maybe our time is tight because we need to revisit our priorities. I don't need to spend as much (or any) time on the Internet—I can neaten up my house. Maybe there's a TV show or two you can give up in order to go for a walk. I just want to encourage some of you out there to look at your lives: Are you being diligent to cultivate faithfulness? Are you tending the sheep of your life? Don't think that just because your patch in the world isn't flashy, it doesn't serve a greater purpose down the road. What can you trade to shepherd your life better in the area of putting in daily physical activity?

You understand that exercise is important because it helps you use more of the fat you've stored and it builds more than physical stamina, but how do you decide what to do?

## But I Don't Wanna Run A Marathon

Good . . . because I have NO desire to swim in the ocean—there are SHARKS out there!

But that doesn't mean you and I can't choose to do something else.

Now that we've discussed the *why* and *how* of maintaining whatever work-out you choose, we need to figure out the *what* you're going to do when you lace up your fancy new kicks, raggedy shorts, and stained T-shirt. (What? Doesn't every flabby person have at least one or two versions of that outfit?)

One of the things I've loved during this whole process of weight loss is learning how much God loves me for who I am (Ps. 147:11). After all, He created me and made me unique (Ps. 100:3). He didn't save me to make me a clone of anyone else in the church; He saved me so that Jesus could shine through who I am and in due time make me Carole perfected (2 Cor. 3:17–18). Just as He gave me my body parts, as well as the ability to draw, sing and write, He also gave me all the good and bad relationships and history which have made me the person I am today; not only me but also all of the people on this earth. If God is sovereign over everything, then everyone who walks the planet owes his or her uniqueness to Him. As I said before, God even uses the terrible circumstances brought about by the wrongs done to us to make us the people we are. Not that He's the author of sin, but God works it out in our lives for a greater purpose. In the end though, each thing He gives to us or brings into our lives is to either make us more into the image of Christ, or if we're not saved, bring us to salvation through Christ (Job 42:1–6; Rom 5:1–5; Rom. 8:18; John 9:30–39; Acts 16:25–31). Since we're such unique creations, why do we think we have to exercise and work out in identical ways? We can't all be on the latest big-body makeover show. We aren't all going to run the Boston Marathon, or even climb mountains, for that matter. We need to discover what works best for us and do that exercise instead of dropping into the stream of popular culture and doing kettlebells just because the guy on TV says, "Do kettlebells."

If you like to walk, go walking. If climbing stairs trips your trigger, then climb away! If you always wanted to hula-hoop while watching recorded episodes of the Iron Chef then get out your hoop and shake your groove thang. Do anything you like, as long as it's something that gets you going. Let no one be the judge of how you decide to move your body as long

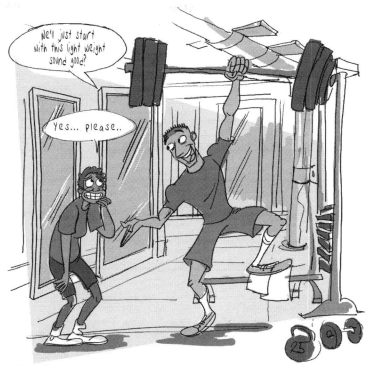

What do you say when a 20 year old jock offers to train you for free?

as you're moving it. Just be faithful to get out there and do it! I think a lot of people give up because they think exercise is too hard. Actually they are the ones who are making it too hard, because they haven't chosen a pastime that suits their preferences and personality. Don't get me wrong, I'm not saying you're going to be doing somersaults down the church aisle because you feel so good doing jumping jacks. What I am saying is that if you find something you actually don't *hate,* you'll be more likely to keep doing it.

When I first started jogging, I didn't love it, but my body did. It wasn't so much that I hated it, but that I was just not good at it. However, it seemed that jogging, no matter how slowly I did it, made the pounds meeeelt awaaaaay. Eventually I realized I enjoyed jogging, and even when I don't want to do anything else, I'll still go out and at least do that. You need to decide what floats your boat when it comes to working out. Because once you do, it'll be easier to get out there and do your twenty-one days without feeling as though you've committed to hit yourself over the head with a hammer until you get in the habit of liking it.

Sometimes the most difficult amount of weight to lift is your own body weight to get up from your chair and get out of the door, so don't make it more difficult by strapping an anvil to your ankle in the form of an exercise you can't stand.

Am I making a case for working out where the Bible is largely silent... well, yes. Let me add this: though whether or not you work out is not evidence of your salvation, it does indicate to what extent you're willing to cede the control of your life to God by maintaining your body so it's able to serve Him well. There are those who look askance at over-spiritualizing everything in our lives. They claim God doesn't care about certain things, only important stuff like sharing the gospel or serving in the church. They don't realize that they unwittingly keep corners of their lives away from the rule of God.

Yet the God who said, *"Go out and preach the gospel to the ends of the earth"* (Matt. 28:19) is the same one who told the apostle Paul to remind us to glorify God with our bodies (1 Cor. 6:19–20).

I'm not saying we're meant to allow this command to make us focus on making our bodies beautiful according to the latest Photohopped covers in the end-cap magazine rack. I'm reminding you that God actually bought our bodies too, not just our souls that ride around in them. Therefore, there's no part of your life over which He hasn't control. He owns ALL of you.

Christ has saved us and calls us to follow Him to the glory of God in *all* areas. Though we struggle, through Jesus we find forgiveness and safety with the Father, who knows we're weak creatures. Let me encourage you excel still more; even if it's at a snail's pace and not a cheetah's run. The world is watching, and though they may insist they want perfection from you now, because "Christians are such hypocrites when they fail," in the long run, those who mock will eventually marvel at a Christian who perseveres in the small things even though it's difficult (1 Pet 2:11–12). I've seen this happen in my life, as the same non-Christian friends who scoff at God are forced to acknowledge my faith when they see how my obedience to Him produces visible change.

As I said before, you are God's gospel tract to your watching world. Therefore, don't underestimate the power your decision to commit to exercise might have to change someone's view of the reality of God. If you can't run three miles, then walk three miles. If you can't walk three miles, then walk one. Eventually this exhaustion will pass, and you'll find new energy on the other side of your slow-motion crawl. But don't give up! Keep. Doing. Something.

## Renewing Your Weakness Renews Your Gratitude

Once you get in the habit of doing some form of exercise, you'll discover you need to push yourself to advance. When I first started, walking was enough to get my heart rate up, and in time I advanced to a slow jog. After a while I needed a bigger challenge than that. I haven't got any really super-spiritual insight to give you as a reason to push yourself continually, except maybe one I had after a recent run:

Continually pushing yourself to do better helps you remember just how weak you are. As you look back at your life traveling from glory to glory in physical activity it gives you the chance to thank God for your progress. The book of Psalms has many calls to remember the deeds of the Lord and find thankfulness in them (Pss. 77:11–13; 78:1–4; 105:1–6; 111:1–4; 143:5). Especially in our Western culture where everything is easy because of technology or even just cars, we need to be constantly reminded that we are not the reason for our greatness, but God is.

Gratitude springs from the understanding that our neediness has been met by someone else's compassionate intervention. When we view our lives as something we can handle, we only have ourselves to thank. Sadly we forget that getting into the car and getting to work is a miracle every day, that at night when we lay our heads on our pillows, it's an act of grace. Believe it or not, I've been constantly reminded that God sustains me because I keep putting myself in challenging positions. Every time I push myself to work out a little harder, I literally pray for the strength and endurance. When I look back on my progress I remember how weak I was and thank Him for helping me be stronger.

I find reasons to be grateful as I'm reminded by my weakness. All the way back when I first started, I wouldn't have repented of greed and gluttony if it weren't for God's revelation. Other people have disputed me on that, telling me I am a strong person or have a great deal of willpower. In that, they try to rob me of the opportunity to be grateful to God and they rob Him of His glory. But the opinions of other people don't matter in the end; what matters is what God did. I know I would be a fat lazy slob if it weren't for His intervention.

# Coasting Doesn't Mean Stopping

If you've picked up this book because you've been working on your weight for a while and you're feeling a little dry; let me encourage you. Recognize that at times you're at the mercy of your human limitations: you might have to scale back for a little while. Unless a radioactive spider has bitten you, normal people don't become superheroes just because they decide to start working out. It's part the curse of Adam. He didn't need no radioactive spider before the Fall, but for us post-Fall people, face it, our body's just wearing out day by day (2 Cor. 4:16). The trick is not to give up completely which is the temptation when one gets tired.

When I was training for my Mount Whitney hike I became a machine. I was running, going to a personal trainer, hiking every week, and even did a half marathon. Then about a month before the hike my body said, "Thanks for playing, have a nice day!"It was like the nightmares I had as a child in which I was being chased by Frankenstein. Though I was running as hard as I could, I was still running in slow motion! It was agony. While it helped my motivation that I was still facing the daunting challenge of having the mountain to climb, a greater thing than the mountain inspired me to push on; my vision of Christ's testimony to a watching world.

It's fabulous to have huge goals but not everyone has time to achieve them. What if you're a mom whose main goal for the moment is raising a family of five, or you're a person who has to work two jobs just to make ends meet? What's to keep you going, even if it's just a little bit? The same thing that kept me going when I didn't have the mountain ahead: my testimony of Christ's transformative love. Remembering that I'm no longer my own because I was bought with a price, so even if I'm tired, giving up completely is no option. This is why the gospel is so important. This is why it's also important to remember why we started dealing with this sin and all the facets of faith that motivate the pursuit of sanctifying our appetites.

This course you're on is not a race against others; it's your life. No one's judging you if you don't get in shape by any set time . . . Well, they may, but who cares? If you're working out to God's glory, the fact that you get up and do something to spend your fat beyond your everyday chores is what's pleasing. If you look in the book of Proverbs, God constantly indicts the sluggard, but I don't see any judgment about the one who is slow but persistent. In fact, God encourages persistence in Proverbs 13:4, *"The soul of the sluggard craves and gets nothing, but the soul of the diligent is made fat."*

In this, we could all stand to put on a little fat in our souls.

## Emotional Weight

*But You, O Lord, are a shield about me, my glory, and the One who lifts my head.*
*I was crying to the Lord with my voice, and He answered me from His holy mountain.*

*Ps. 3:3*

One last encouragement for anyone starting exercise or trying to find motivation to keep going when you aren't one of those people who just looooves doing it. Though sometimes it's simple laziness that prevents us from reprioritizing our lives so that exercise plays a part in it—sometimes it might also be because we're emotionally hurting. It can be difficult to lift your body if your soul is heavy with sorrow, frustration, loneliness, anxiety or fear. As I wrote in my blog regarding such a time:

> *I've been looking for the past two weeks and have lost all motivation to do anything (which is strange since I started this whole odyssey when I was unemployed). The issue here is not physical exhaustion, but emotional paralysis . . . I sat down before the Lord and told Him how I felt: sad, lonely, scared. I waited, silent and tearful. After a bit of time I took a look at all that was going on in my heart and realized that all those emotions I was feeling were like a seemingly normal patch of grass covering a deadly punji pit filled with spikes! The emotions were covering my disbelief of truths about God's gracious character!*

As long as we live, we'll be in a constant battle between expectations and reality, and the siege is a wearing one. While sometimes the emotions are caused by wrongs we experience, other times they spring from our inability to accept the circumstances in our lives as ones God means for us to have. Either way I'm not saying it's bad to feel bad, but what do you do once you acknowledge how badly you feel? Where do you go to deal with those feelings? We need to turn to God, who is sovereign over everything and who knows your thoughts and emotions. The God we serve isn't in the business of saving us and leaving us to struggle alone (Phil. 1:6; 1 Thess. 5:23–24).

God wants to be your emotional "spotter." If you've been at a gym, you know what I mean. You've seen those guys who lift giant weights, with their buddy standing over them to help them raise the bar after they've done a bunch of repetitions and their arms are Jello but they still need to put the barbell back to its resting place. While in spotting you, God may not remove the weighty circumstance, He who knows the muscles of character that you're building will help you bear the burden of your heavy heart—if you don't give up and lose hope. Just cry out to Him in raw honesty that you need His help!

# Emancipated Angels

*For the Lord takes pleasure in His people; He will beautify the afflicted ones with salvation.*

*Ps. 149:4*

Yes, God cares about our insecurities, struggles and hurts. In light of that let me address the idea that God is only concerned about the heart, while man focuses on the outside.

Just because Jesus was an unremarkable-looking man, and the apostles were never described doesn't mean that God doesn't care how you feel about your looks. He does tell us not to focus on them because they can be surfacy and vain if your character is out of whack (1 Pet. 3:3–4; Prov. 31:30) but that doesn't mean He doesn't care about how you feel about yourself.

God shows that He is capable of sympathy for our insecurities about our self-image by the simple fact that He included the issue in the Song of Solomon. When Solomon's new bride felt insecure about her looks compared to others, he tells her in no uncertain terms that he thinks she's beautiful. From then on, she never brings up her insecurities about her looks again, as she focuses on how beautiful he is (Song 1:5–6; 8–9).

God sees your heart. He knows you compare yourself to others around you, and yet to Him you are beautiful and so are they. Why? Because He created you.

The you that you see in the mirror: That is who you are. It's so much more than ectomorph/endomorph, pear- or apple-shaped. All the dimples are yours. The ratio of shoulders to waist to hips, those are yours and yours alone. Sure, long after you lose the weight, effects of the sin of gluttony may remain: the sags and squish. But beneath it all, this is who God made you to be (Ps. 139:13–16).

As an artist, I delight in the characters I create. I put thought and effort into giving them characteristics that I think serve to tell others a little bit about them. Shouldn't God, who's infinite and endlessly creative, do the same thing with real people? While there are times when the effects of sin, whether disease or abuse, do mar God's designs for humans, it's only man in his sin who has taken the elements of design God has given each person and turned them into reasons to worship or ostracize each other.

There's peace to be found when we understand that God designed our bodies the way He did because our crooked toes, big or little noses, hair that cowlicks, awkward double-jointed limbs or any host of anatomical affects was intentionally and intelligently done to suit His purpose (Ex. 4:10–11; Job 33:4; Ps. 100:3; Ps. 139:13–16; Isa. 44:24; John 1:3; Col. 1:16–17).

In light of that understanding I set about uncovering the physique God gave uniquely to me. Michelangelo is reputed to have said of his sculptures: "I saw an angel in the marble and I set it free." When I first started losing weight, I was intrigued by that idea because a friend who's as lithe as a panther told me his athletic anatomy was genetic. Later I met a

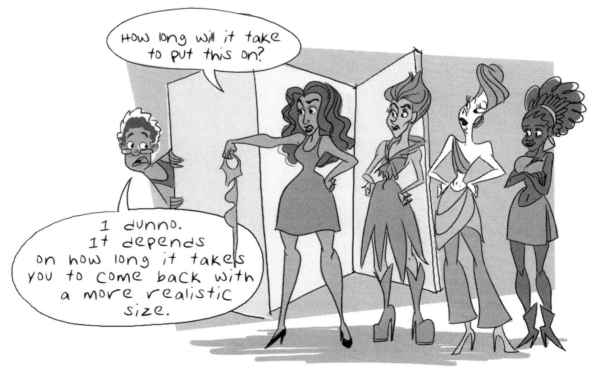

why I'll never have a career as a model

woman who grumbled at my innocent question of how much time she spent in the gym. She replied with a terse, "None…I was just born with man arms." I was excited as I wondered what lay under all this body fat?

Well five years later I realized that this is it. It's neither athletic nor perfectly proportioned. Some parts are big when they could be smaller and some parts are smaller when maybe they could be a *little bit* bigger. I may not have man arms or a panther body but this is mine and mine alone.

You and I are the way we are because God imagined us to be this way. I may or may not be beautiful to some, but to God I'm delightful because He's an artist, and don't all artists like what they make and put on display?

Let that change your perspective on working out. Remember God, your Creator, thinks you're beautiful because He made you, so focus your praise on Him who loves you. Rejoice in the fact that you don't have to prove anything to others by improving your hotness quotient by working out, because you're already a work of art. Your fat is covering the handiwork God made to be displayed to give Him glory as a designer and it is the equivalent to putting ugly scaffolding around Michelangelo's David. Get that stuff outta there. To the best of your ability, let those all around you see the Creator's creation in you.

# Though You May Toss Your Cookies, It Will Eventually End

There's something beautiful in how each of us is made, both inside and outside. Yes, we could all work out like fiends until we looked like those people from any of the body makeover shows—but why, really? I mean if you really want to, then go for it, but most people struggle with just exercising at all without adding the thought that they are going to have to be an example of what a human can look like at their peak. Muscles were designed for a purpose, just like storing fat was designed for a purpose; it's us who've elevated them to a status symbol. Any created thing can easily become a source of worship (or of finding a way to bring us worship). We need to remember that and also remember that the purpose of having a well-functioning body is to be able to serve God in everything He gives us to do with all the strength we have.

With these words, I'm not advocating that you stop doing all your household duties and family obligations so you can get pumped in the gym. What I'm encouraging you in this chapter of "Do" is to commit to purposefully do what you can to steadily use the resources you've stored so that you can train your body to live for God's glory. I know it's challenging, but the praise you're able to give God when others ask you why have you changed is far more worth it than the latest made-for-streaming Internet original mini series, or anything else for that matter.

I spent the autumn at cross-country meets watching my young friend do what she does exceptionally well: run. Whenever she runs the course she literally does the whole thing with a smile and crosses the finish line near the front of the pack as she tries each time to do better than the last. The thing is though, most of the time she also crosses the finish line and throws up. One day I asked her how she can run so hard that clearly her body is in pain and she replied, "Because I know it's just a little bit and then it will be over."

In this life there are so many races we must run and they can be like cross-country meets, which are harder because the terrain is uneven and while there may be flat straight places, there are also hills with which to contend. In being faithful to exercise, we receive more than better health and an effective way of burning fat. We can learn faithfulness in just lacing up a pair of kicks every day, and that may train us for greater challenges. Or we may see that in our weakness God will give us what we need to face anything, from trials from the world to overcoming internal struggles.

Just remember, this race of life is little in the light of eternity and one day it will end, so while it may hurt for a while, the pain of the struggle cannot compare to the relief and prize of having run the race to the best of your ability. So put on your shoes and get out there!

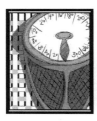

# Take A-Weigh

- View exercise as making good on your promise you made when you ate all that food.
- Cultivating faithfulness in mundane and small things like daily exercise prepares you for whatever God has planned for you.
- Just do ANYTHING to get started. As you see progress, challenge yourself to do more.
- There are benefits to exercising beyond getting in better shape physically.
- While God is not preoccupied with your appearance, He does care about your insecurities regarding your looks.
- God will be your Comforter when you need Him; don't give up.

# Food for Thought

*"Commit your works to the Lord and your plans will be established."* Proverbs 16:3

My best good friend jokes that she goes to the gym because the Proverbs 31 woman "girded herself with strength and made her arms strong . . ." (Prov. 31:17). Whether or not that's the perfect practical application for that verse, I admire my friend because she's as purposeful in choosing to exercise as she is caring for her house, her husband's business, and her children, whom she homeschools. Finding time to move your arms and legs can be done.

No one is asking you to train like a triathlete. Just pick something simple and doable, then *purposefully make it a part of your day* like you schedule your dinner menus, clean your house, or pick up your kids from school.

"It's all a matter of priorities," a young friend of mine once said as we finished a leisurely six-mile hike. "If you're physically capable, there's always something that can give in your schedule to make room for a little exercise." She was six months pregnant and holding the hand of her two-year-old daughter at the time.

- **What are your excuses for not exercising, beyond that it hurts and you hate it?**

- **What can you give up in your day to incorporate purposeful exercise?**

- **What exercises do you like to do?**

- **What's your best time of day to exercise?**

- **Do you have friends or family with whom to exercise?**

- **Choose three days a week in which to do twenty minutes of your favorite exercise.**

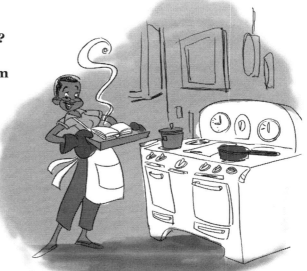

Because no one ever gained a pound from thinking too much.

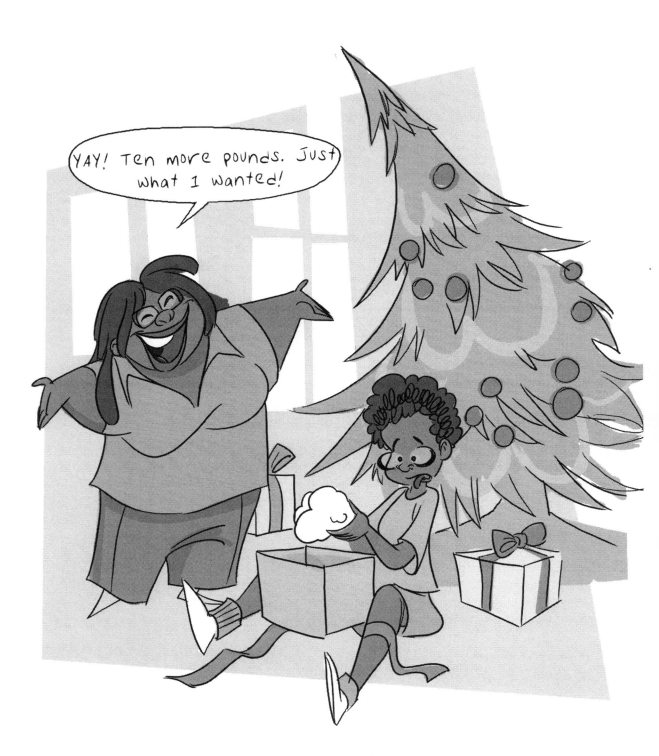

Unhappy Holliday...

Chapter 12

# Don't Hate What You Ate

> *Act as free men, and do not use your freedom as a covering for evil, but use it as bondslaves of God.*
> *2 Pet. 2:16*

My friend was far too beautiful to look like your typical animator; she looked more like a model. Animation people can be awkward. They're a mixture of actor and wallflower, incredible exhibitionists who'd rather hide in the shadows. Not her. As she slipped into a slinky blue velvet dress for the Hercules® wrap party, she and I were an unlikely pair—she was like a gazelle and I . . . well, I was more like a hippo who sat with an awkward kerplop on a tiny chair outside the dressing room. As she tousled her auburn hair, pouted her lips, and sized herself up in the mirror, I thought how wonderful it would be to look like her.

Within the next year, she discovered she was pregnant. Now you think I'm going to tell you that she blew up like a puffer fish. No. She didn't. She stayed small, and is almost as small today, two children and ten years later. She still looks hot. So this isn't a story about size: It's a story about appetite. One day my pregnant friend talked about the changes her body was going through and said with alarm, "I just ate a whole foot-long sandwich!"

"Yes?" I replied.

"A whole one!"

She was appalled. She'd never done that before. To her it was enormous.

To her. Really?

I was silent . . .

To me that was normal.

It was normal for me to eat a foot-long submarine sandwich. With chips. . . . and a drink. That would have been light, actually.

There was a neighborhood burger joint that had the best french fries. So I always got two . . . in addition to the double chili cheeseburger and orange soda. I didn't discriminate between different food nationalities. I loved them all the same. I could never make up my mind at my favorite Mexican taco stand. Should it be the burrito, the torta, or the tacos? Okay, how about all of them . . . at once. Two pizzas—not slices, entire ones—well, at least they were mediums. I could polish off a plate of lamb kebab, two or three cups of rice, several pitas, a salad, and half a dozen nazook pastries, as well as various other Armenian cookies. My appetite was endless and writing this now, my eyes well up with tears as I think of the person that I once was. The apostle Paul describes some as people whose *god is their appetite* and whose *end is destruction* (Phil. 3:19). I was one of those, and the shame is that I did it while claiming to be under the ownership of Jesus Christ!

Anyone who continues to live with unchecked passions needs to consider whether or not they're putting themselves under the Shepherd's staff. If they're truly saved, He's a loving protector who won't let them stray for long. How long it is, though, I cannot say.

All I know is that God made it abundantly clear He wasn't going to stand my gluttony any longer. Yes, there was a health scare, but I'd had those before. It was more than that—I can't describe it any better than to say it was an impending sense that He was going to bring the hammer down and it wasn't going to be just a slap on the wrist. The warning was loud and clear: "Repent of your rebellion, or else." I have often written across the pages of this book about the love of God—but I have also said a loving Father disciplines, too. There came a time when God made it apparent to me that He was demanding every part of me, down to the food I put in my mouth, and He wanted me to do something more than diet. Dieting attacks only the effects with its restriction of calories and demonization of certain foods. I'd dieted before, but every time I ate a "bad" food, I'd throw up my hands and go back to my wicked, wicked ways because I didn't see the problem as God saw it: The type of food I ate wasn't the culprit that spread my hips and obscured my eyes with mountains of fat, it was the amount.

I've spoken about God's discipline because of my experience. I could tell I was under His heavy hand and yet once I came to repentance and knelt before Him with a trembling heart at 312 pounds, I discovered God's loving freedom and grace. God demanded that I quit making food an idol but He also showed me that He didn't want me to run from what I ate but instead be thankful for it, to take what I needed to satisfy me, and move on.

I learned I could eat anything . . .

Really?

Yes, child . . . anything (Col. 2:16–23).

From there, that's how I changed the way that I ate. Believe it or not: the first three months of testing this newfound freedom in Christ, I ate burgers, fries, cakes and pies and lost thirty pounds—but I ate less of them!

He had my attention: God, in His kindness, showed me He could be trusted. From there He led me by the hand into the dark and oftentimes rocky places of my heart to help me clean the clutter of my covetous soul. He trained my arms to bend the bow of bronze to make my appetite my slave and not the other way around. He gave me a means to have more success than failures. And when I did fail, He gave me the means to find my way back to the path from which I had strayed. This book contains some of the things He's shown me.

At first I didn't know all of the things I'm sharing with you in the pages of this book; I discovered His tender promises across the battlefields of my will along the way. My understanding of obeying God in regard to my appetite has evolved since I first repented, but in this chapter I'll talk about eating.

I could tell you how I chose to eat—and in fact, I will—but I do it with this admonition: Be careful not to turn my suggestions into a set of laws. Manmade laws do nothing to restrict the longings of the heart. If anything, they cause it to boil over somewhere else. Merely "doing good" is not enough, in the end you need to be transformed from your heart, and that may take a lifetime.

# The Basis for My Biblical Eating

We're all interested in watching what we eat and how much we move or else we wouldn't be here, right? We read the labels. We watch the clocks to figure out how long we've been at our jogs, our walks, and our slow trudges through the neighborhood. We rejoice at the numbers as they tick off on the treadmill telling us we've burned the amount of calories—just UNDER the piece of cake we ate yesterday after church.

The best advice I can give you in this battle of your belly is to stop trying to lose weight. Instead make it your goal to be obedient to God in what you know to be true regarding your eating. That's what I did. I did it even though I didn't feel like doing it. I did it at first because I thought if I believe there is a God who rules my life, I needed to obey Him for the sake of obeying. The weight I subsequently lost was the bonus off to the side.

Through the pages of this book I've discussed the theology that propelled me in my obedience to God in the area of my appetite.

1. God wanted me to have a submitted appetite instead of dieting (1 Sam. 15:22).

2. Food wasn't the demon; my greedy heart was (Mark 7:14–23).

3. No food was a bad food (Acts 10:9–15).

4. I needed to cultivate an attitude of thankfulness for the food God gave me instead of making it a god (Rom. 1:25).

5. I needed to eat to glorify God instead of myself (1 Cor. 10:31).

6. I needed to apply the things I already knew in regard to eating (James 4:17).

7. I needed to be content with the time it took to show results from obeying God (Prov. 19:2).

The Bible is a mirror of God that shows us our flaws in comparison to God's holiness. The Bible helped me understand what I'm basically saying when I choose to overindulge: "I want to be in charge of my life, not God." When I do this, I'm no better than the evil villain referred to in Isaiah 14:13-14 who sought to exalt himself above God.

I know I'm not alone; we all do this in some form or another when we insist on continuing in our beloved sins. Just as the character in Isaiah's proud assumptions began and ended with the pronoun "I" so do we when we insist "My way is better than God's way for me."

While ceasing to be greedy is our goal so that we won't keep fueling our fat cells and instead start using the fat that's in them. If we don't deal with the underlying attitudes that can cause us to eat, we'll fall prey to our own friendly fire; while we're seeking to put down the fork with one hand, our heart will be grabbing for the bag of salty snacks with the other. Over the years I've been on this journey, I've learned there were four fronts I have to be vigilant about if I wanted to check my propensity to eat sinfully: Impatience, Ingratitude, Indecision and Intractability.

- I'll have it now.
- I'll have it all.
- I'm not happy with what I have. / I want *more* of what I have.
- I want things the way I want them.

# I'll Have It Now

*Impatience wants it now.*

I spoke about patience in chapter 8. Here I'll talk about his bizarro cousin *"Im*-patience". In eating, the practical application for patience is to slow down. How often was I impatient, the first person done at the dinner table. How often are you? We need to quit being impatient and eat the things set before us more slowly, whether it's sugar snap peas or pizza.

The benefit in patiently eating is that you allow your body to experience being satisfied. I suppose appetite satiety is different for everyone, but it's something each of us needs to learn and get used to; just as we need to get used to the habit of exercising. Otherwise when we're outside of our home where we can control our meals—at parties, or fancy restaurants, or if we eventually marry someone who has a different idea of what food is "safe" to have around the house—then we can undo everything we did!

While it would be nice if everyone understood the struggles we have in our gluttony and that the world just "got" that they need to give us only what we needed, in the end, it's up to us to learn to control our appetite.

Patience is a step toward training ourselves to be satisfied. Impatience is the enemy of learning that lesson.

Not only do we need to be patient to learn the lesson of personal satiety, we also need to not be impatient for results from our obedience. I know if you're like me, you hesitate to start losing weight because it takes so long to do it. There are so many things God longs to give us that are more lasting than a better body. So repent of your impatience and need for speed and learn to value the time as God's gift to truly do what He wants accomplished in your life.

You look at extreme weight loss shows and it's easy to be impressed with the fast weight loss, but who gets the glory for it? You thought I was going to say the contestants. No. The show does. Just look at the testimonials. All they say is "This show changed my life!" When I started down this road of obedient eating, I didn't want to say that. I didn't want to say any diet program or anything other than God changed my life. I wanted to be able to say that I believe in God so much that I'm willing to give Him control of everything; even the power over my eating. Not only did He give me forgiveness and the hope of eternal life; He is renovating this broken-down life and turning it into something beautiful.

I know, to many, it's just a matter of semantics. But the thing is, those TV shows and diet programs will go away, but God is eternal. God is also gracious; much more than the giant unforgiving scale each contestant has to face at the end of the week, or in the program that you dread as you're scanning the shelves for some other diet aid you hope might make the difference next week. In diets, the reward is the final number on the scale, with the winning coming only when you've hit that magic number. In God, winning isn't the results the world can see; but the submitted obedience to Him. Every meal I ate to His glory was a victory, so every meal where I chose to obey Him was where I could find success. With each act of obeying Him, God saw me as having already reached my goal, the weight wasn't the issue: submitted obedience to His rule in my life was. When we cease being impatient for the big results and content ourselves with the results that God thinks are important, He grows our character (Ps. 51:6–7; 2 Cor. 4:16–18; Eph. 3:14–19; Col. 3:1–10).

Often when we look at what's in front of us to accomplish, it seems like a big ton of work that's going to take forever so we either don't want to do it or we try to find short cuts to get to what we think is the end. We need to understand that though you may seem to be left with tedious tasks while you're waiting for your results, actually patiently persevering in those tasks will prepare you for something greater than your goal. We have such a tiny picture of our lives. We just want to lose weight, but God wants us to be transformed into the image of Christ—He's got bigger plans, beyond our smaller belt size. So repent of your impatience, trust the time it takes to achieve sanctification in any area God calls you to submit to Him, and do this all the while remembering each act of obedience is the victory!

## I'll Have It All

*Indecision can't make up its mind which one to choose.*

Another contributing factor to long-term weight gain is indecisiveness. This, coupled with greed, creates a perfect storm that plays out in our eating—because if we're indecisive we won't narrow our food choice to one option. In the end, we don't make a choice—we take it all.

We talked about faithfulness in the previous chapter, however people who are indecisive can be like the faithless man (Prov. 25:19) because their lack of decisiveness about submitting their appetites to be governed by God's commands indicates that their character shouldn't be trusted.

The definition of faithless in the Hebrew equates it to being treacherous: like a rocky path on a steep mountain trail. I learned to be cautious when walking on a steep rocky trail because I couldn't be certain that the rocks I stepped on were not going to shift. Likewise, indecisive people show a character that can't be relied upon because it can be changed by circumstances or emotions.

James 1:8 says a double-minded man is unstable in all his ways. So your inability to choose and find satisfaction in your choice betrays a greater problem than whether you took the pie and cake.

When I was elephantine, I never made choices. Whether it was from fear, dissatisfaction, covetousness or just plain laziness. I always left it to someone else to decide. "What are you getting?" I'd say as I polled my friends at a restaurant, or "let me get back to you," I'd innocently reply if I received an invitation to an event, making sure I had a chance to scan the online list of who was going to the party before I'd give a yes or no.

We're all guilty of it in one form or another, but we need to put a stop to it as one of the many bad habits that keep us from losing weight. We need to learn to choose and let the chips fall where they may. God is in control of our life, but He's given us the amazing gift of free will. So many of us abnegate that gift by our indecisiveness or use it against God when we tell Him, "No, thank you very much." If God wants us to give control of our lives to Him, even to the extent of putting food in our bellies, then let us partner with Him to use our gift of free will to conscientiously decide what goes in there.

If you struggle with indecision, then try an experiment for a month. Actually make a choice. If presented with several food options, choose one. This experiment isn't permanent, but try it for a time, until you master your appetite.

Learning to make decisions in your food will affect other areas of your life. There's a notion that if you struggle with a particular sin in one area, you will struggle with it in all areas of your life. For example: I refused to be self-controlled in my eating, and it was no surprise that my house was a disaster, my finances were tenuous, and I was even carefree about my speed on the freeway. So when I started working on submitting to God's will regarding self-control in eating, I worked hard to do it in all areas of my life.

When I realized I needed to be decisive about my food choices, I understood I needed to the same in other areas of my life. So when I started cleaning my cluttered house I forced myself to make a decision about everything I touched. Oftentimes I'd discover I had several of the same type of items. Whether it was vintage radios, antique clocks or several mismatched sets of silverware; I chose my favorite one and parted with the duplicates. It wasn't easy, because I had to fight with the sentimental value I'd placed on things—but that's for another book . . . The main point is: Working on being decisive meant in the end that I had a clutter-free home.

I'm not saying you have to go around having one of each thing for the rest of your life. This is where moderation comes in. Of course you still have to live, but in the case of those occasional events where you're not being indecisive but actually *do want to sample several items,* exercise portion control and take less of both.

So many times when faced with indecision we not only choose both, but we choose both as though they were "the only." We get the whole giant slice of aunt Flo's once-a-year pound cake and an entire piece of Grandmother Jemma's killer cherry pie. If you have exhibited decisive moderation and you find there's something you'd rather have more of, ask if you can have some to enjoy later rather than trying to eat it all now. Be more purposeful. Decide whether to go left or right, forward or backward, to have a burrito or a taco. Learn to choose and you'll find stability, peace and confidence as you grow in your identity Christ; you'll see that your decisions, as dedicated to the glory of God, matter.

# The Insatiable Appetite

*Ingratitude is never satisfied and always wants something different.*

Even if we manage to be patient to wait for results and cultivate decisiveness and faithfulness, becoming trustworthy as a result, we can undermine it all by being ungrateful. Gluttons generally don't take the time to be thankful even that we have food in the first place. Jesus said that God would provide our needed food, just as He provides it for the birds (Matt. 6:25–26). Since that's the case, we should be grateful for the food that we get because the beneficent, almighty God who keeps the world in motion has interacted with us even in the simple act of getting a burger.

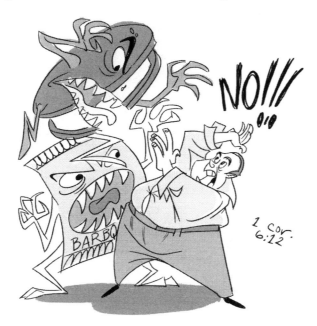

"All things are lawful for me, but not all things are profitable. All things are lawful for me, but I will not be mastered by anything."

When is the last time you were genuinely grateful for what's on your plate in front of you? When were you grateful for all that went to get from the field or farm to the table with skill (or at least with love, if you're chef's not such a great cook)?

Instead of turning the holidays with family and friends into an excuse for food orgies we need to even be grateful for eating with those people we love; after all, we could have everything we desire and still be miserable (Prov. 15:17). In all things, we need to see each meal as God's gracious provision to help those of us with greedy proclivities to go from being greedy gobblers to grateful grubbers!

We miss out on the magnificent revelation of God's interaction with His lowly creatures because we mindlessly, thanklessly gobble, gobble, gobble. We need to purposefully take time to slow down and see what's right in front of us. It may seem strange, but something that helped me begin to see what I had in front of me so that I could be grateful was actually taking the time to look at my food before I shoveled it into my mouth.

I learned to eat with my eyes before I ate with my mouth.

There was a point in the evolution of social media when people were constantly posting pictures of their meals. Not just any meal, but their fancy desserts, delicious breads and gorgeous plates. Why not do the same with your everyday meals? Except not on Facebook. Here's another experiment for you, based on the concept of social media's obsession with food ("food porn"). For a month, take pictures of your meals before you eat them. Your bowl of breakfast oatmeal and banana, your plate of pasta primavera with prawns, your bag of airplane peanuts or your cup of coffee and scone: whatever you're eating, display it pleasantly and snap a picture of it.

When I'd photograph my meals (sending them to someone for a time in accountability) it did two things, it helped my accountability partner see what I was eating and it actually helped me see what I was eating. This was three years into eating rightly. However before my food photo experiment, even though I was choosing to eat decisively and in the right amounts, I still felt like I wasn't getting enough food. I realized it was in my head. Taking the time to organize my portions on the plate and even thinking about where it came from helped me to think, *Oh my goodness, I get all this food? And it's good? Wow, God, you're so kind!*

It's by no means a permanent way to live your life, always arranging and taking pictures of your food, but it's good training for your brain that's used to seeing things in drips and dribbles. (Or not at all, if you're eating in front of a television or computer screen.) Take time to see your food and you'll learn to see how blessed you are.

People are larger today than they were in my grandparent's generation; I don't know if it's because of fast food, abundant food, or not seeing your food. I just know that for me, the times I actually focus on a meal are more satisfying than the times I'm eating as an afterthought. In bygone times, when people used to sit down and eat meals with one another and people don't seem to have been as fat as they are now, they enjoyed their meal in the company of those they loved but then moved on to clear off the table. No wonder we don't have gratitude for our meals, since we're quickly grabbing a bite here while looking the other way, or snacking out of dark crinkly bags, or standing grazing from the fridge, or mindlessly swallowing everything on our plates like snakes when they unhinge their jaws to gobble down bunnies.

*Yick.*

We need to take the time to take those food pictures even if they're just mental ones. We need to see the provision right before us and appreciate it.

Above all as Christians, we should be the most thankful people on the planet because, despite any of our circumstances—whether we're rich or poor, alone or in a relationship, whether we can afford sushi or only cans of tuna—God has saved us (John 6:37). We know God answers our prayers (Col. 4:2) and though everything we love on this earth my fall away, we have the promise of an eternal Kingdom (Heb. 12:28). In the simple act of eating, we can learn to practice gratitude that goes beyond the mechanical routine of saying grace over meals, because we know the God who provided those meals. *We know Him!*

# I Want Things the Way I Want Them

*The intractable person just won't be content in life as God gives it to them.*

Overeating is a form of control. When situations are distasteful we look for things that are tasty to make something pleasant in our lives. But we need to cease running from the disappointments of our lives, because they actually have a purpose—strengthening us. I've mentioned before the notion that God takes everything in our lives, the acts of obedience and situations that happen to us, and works it together to make us into the image of Christ. God uses everything—the good, the bad, and the indifferent circumstances—as ingredients for a recipe to bake us into the people He wants us to be.

The distasteful elements in our lives are just as important as the sweet, tasty moments, much as baking soda and salt have an awful taste on their own yet without them, the recipe falls flat and lacks depth. We need to come to God in prayer that He would quiet our hearts regarding the foul-tasting morsels of our lives. Then we can recognize that they do have a purpose; we can find the savor of sweetness, not in the circumstances themselves, but in the Maker of the circumstances. He understands His recipe for each of us.

It is often said that God works all things for His glory and our good, but *what's that good?* It isn't always a better situation down the road. It may not be a promotion in the next job when you got fired unjustly from your last, nor a hot spouse when the person you pined for falls in love with someone else, nor even a family who adopts you when your family of origin has rejected you. It may not be any of the many dreams you long for when your heart is broken and your spirit is crushed by rejection and loss. We need to see what's really "good" as our heavenly Father sees it. God's plans for our good are far loftier than our weak eyes can see on earth. His ultimate plan is to return this world to what it once was—a place where He walked with His creation in a time before the fall of man (Rev. 22:1–5). For the Christian, this is the bittersweet joy in the "no's" of life—each "no" is a "yes" in Him.

We need to fight like the dickens to remember this; we need to put our faith in the One who controls everything instead of turning to food to control *something*. It's a hard battle to remember the truth of God's ultimate plan as opposed to the reality of that chocolate you can see and scarf down when you're not hungry. The chocolate is truly the lie—not God.

I don't want to be a cold-hearted ogre about this, because I know what it feels like. At times I've sought to control something in my life by eating; I'm genuinely hurting because my dreams were crushed or I'm really scared because my life seems out of control for the moment. We truly can be driven to the sin of greed because we're in pain. However, we need to remind ourselves of the truth in those times of temptation: God is sovereign in the painful

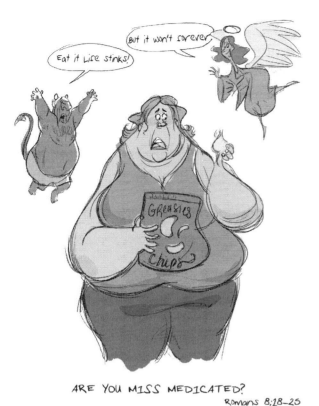

ARE YOU MISS MEDICATED?
Romans 8:18–25

circumstances that happen in our lives, though He doesn't cause our sin, and He uses those trials to expose the weaknesses in our character so He can fix them in preparation for our eternal lives with Him.

So while it doesn't decrease the agony of our disappointments, we can take comfort in the overall purpose of pain. For us as individuals who are waiting for our final rest in a pain-free eternity with Christ, our pain should serve as an alarm to indicate the weakness in our character, like a creak in a rotten floorboard alerts a person to a potentially painful consequence.

When such a weakness is uncovered, we have two choices: find temporary (and often self-destructive) comfort in ourselves through control, or run to God for comfort—meted out in ways we can't foresee—and for His lasting repair. As I write this I'm in great pain over a crushing disappointment. It doesn't matter what it is, but know that it is common to man. In the midst of this pain, I'm reminded that any trial's greatest lesson is to show us that this world is a faulty replacement for a painless heaven. In God's kingdom there will be no sin, in us or around us, and because of that, no pain either.

Remember God has promised to take care of those who are His own and He always keeps His word (Num. 23:19; Titus 1:2; Heb. 6:18). Therefore every circumstance He brings through our lives has a purpose for our sanctifying good—deep down in our heart and character where it really matters. So we need to stop being intractable when He wheels up the dessert-tray of distasteful events: we need to eat the bread of pain in equal measure with the meals that satisfy us and we'll begin to see results not because we dieted them away, but because we aren't stuffing the fat suitcases with stress fat. When we only focus on correcting a behavior, like losing a few pounds we gained because we ate as a form of control, we're merely dealing with the external problem, like putting a Band-Aid® on a sketchy mole.

# God's Plan in Your Repentence

If we are merely seeking to shed some inconvenient habit or even to obey God in transforming some behavior, we're missing the point. The point is not only to be like Him in repentance; the point is to be *with* Him.

Unless we deal with some of the underlying attitudes that cause us to eat, we're only putting a coat of paint over a moldy wall. We need to deal with issues of indecision, impatience, ingratitude, and intractability, or the weight will keep coming back because we haven't cut off the source of our mindless eating. Only God is the answer to all of those heart grumps I've mentioned. Not God plus some program or system of external works, but God Himself.

When Moses asked God, "Who should I say sent me?" God replied "I AM has sent me to you" (Ex. 3:13–14). As I've said before, I'm not a Bible scholar, but an artist. But I take encouragement from what I learned about God while I was working on an animated film about the time of the Hebrews' exodus from Egypt. While doing research, I discovered that the Egyptians had over three hundred gods, gods that were no gods at all: gods of water, air and everything kind of matter. Moses grew up with that mentality. Since that was the case, when he asked that question, I wonder if he was really asking, "Who should I tell them sent me? Are you god #301?"

God unequivocally replied. *I AM.* Meaning He's the God above all others. He's the One who actually exists.

When we merely seek to abolish the consequences of our greed without dealing with the heart beneath it we're in danger of being Moses-minded. We need to repent of those bad attitudes, definitely, but we also need to move beyond simply adding godly things to make our lives better. We need to seek God Himself. This is why it's imperative that you spend as much time running to God as you do running from your former manner way of life. Otherwise when times get tough you will find yourself lashing out at God and running back to your crutch of sin.

Though we may not be physically sightless or need the help of crutches to walk, we greedily eat when we become blinded by the pain of our circumstances, not remembering that heaven is coming, or we seek to prop ourselves up with encouragement from a rich meal when we're feeling poor in our spirits. Jesus came to give sight to the blind and to heal the lame. Turn to Him who will give you eyes to see eternity and feet to run to Him and you will find ways to battle your indecisive, impatient, ungracious and discontented heart.

*When my heart was embittered*
*and I was pierced within,*
*Then I was senseless and ignorant;*
*I was like a beast before You.*
*Nevertheless I am continually with You;*
*You have taken hold of my right hand.*
*With Your counsel You will guide me,*
*and afterward receive me to glory.*
*Whom have I in heaven but You?*
*And besides You, I desire nothing on earth.*
*My flesh and my heart may fail,*
*but God is the strength of my heart and my portion forever.*

Ps. 73:21–26

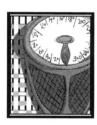

# Take A-Weigh

- All food is good. Just eat LESS of it.
- We can fight our greed by cultivating gratitude, decisiveness, and patience.
- God and God alone is the answer to what causes us to eat greedily.

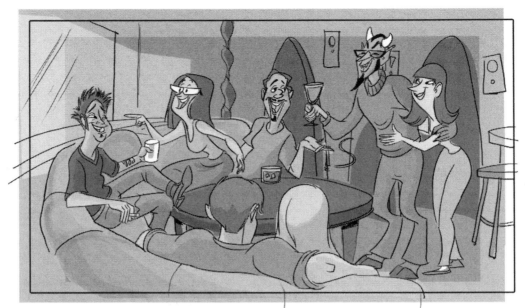

French poet Charles Baudelaire said, "The greatest trick the Devil ever did was convincing the world he did not exist."

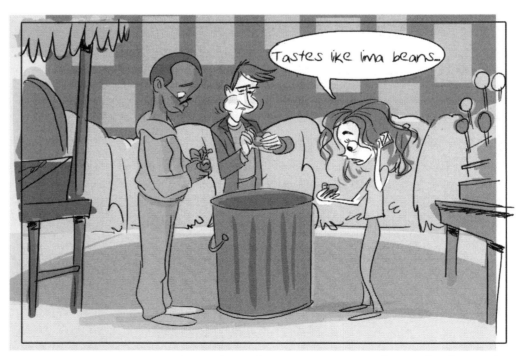

The second greatest one was inspiring the words to the song that made eating chestnuts seem like a great idea.

Chapter 13

# Love the Food You're With

*"Do you not understand that whatever goes into the man from outside cannot defile him, because it does not go into his heart, but into his stomach, and is eliminated?" (Thus He declared all foods clean.) And He was saying, "That which proceeds out of the man, that is what defiles the man. For from within, out of the heart of men, proceed the evil thoughts, fornications, thefts, murders, adulteries, deeds of coveting and wickedness, as well as deceit, sensuality, envy, slander, pride and foolishness. All these evil things proceed from within and defile the man."*     Mark 7:18-23

It's time we stopped blaming the food we consume for our big butts. Not one time in my gluttonous life did my doorbell ring and braised green beans, firecracker shrimp, a tub of won ton soup and steamed pork dumplings lurch across my threshold, slither across the floor, hop up to the dining room table of their own accord and say, "Hey, lets have dinner!"

No, I made those choices. I made those calls. I went to those restaurants and I ate them all!

Blaming any food for our long-term weight gain is disrespectful to the God who created it. When we demonize many foods it's as if we raised our clenched fist to our loving Father and said, "God it's Your fault I'm overweight, that I have diabetes, bad knees and a bad back! You made this food far, far too good!" I know we don't believe that we think that way when we pass on Grandma's secret recipe oyster giblet stuffing because it contains bread, but that's the underlying attitude we have in our heart when we take food, which is morally neutral, and blame it for our external results. God made all the things we love to eat, but we are the ones who turn the fuel He gives us into a form of entertainment. Food by itself is neither good nor bad.

In the end—food just lies there.

Prrrurthch.

See it sitting there on the plate . . . it might be pretty, (or in my case, it might be slightly scorched) but the point is that food isn't the problem. We are.

We're greedy, indecisive, impatient, and ungrateful. We refuse to use the self-control God has given us and we make ourselves slaves to the rush of brain chemicals created as a natural response to the taste of food on our tongues. We realize there's a problem, but we attack the wrong source. Because of our self-deception we subject ourselves to arbitrary restrictions regarding our food intake "I can't eat sugar" or "I can't eat fat" or "I can't eat bread" or . . .

Until the act of eating becomes a chore, or boring, or our master. I don't think that God who created taste buds meant for our food to become just medicine; how cruel would that be? When I realized that food was not the issue but I was, I was faced with standing there guilty and without an excuse before a holy God. No ifs, ands—yet having a great big butt.

Again . . . I'm glad God isn't like me. If I were in His place, I'd reward my guilty verdict with punishment—or at very least with the cold shoulder. Not God, not only did He put the penalty of my guilt on His only begotten beloved Son, God took pity on me as well as anyone who recognizes they're responsible to pay for the sin in their lives and He becomes their helper to overcome their affliction, and their refuge in their weakness. God will never cast out anyone who admits they've failed and that they need His help.

God, our mighty yet merciful benevolent Teacher, has a better way for us regarding eating. Not one that leads to more laws but a way that lets us play like children in fields of food freedom. With Him we can quit making food the devil in the scenario of our burgeoning size: for God wants food to be what it is:

Just food.

And with this realization we can become content (1 Tim. 6:7–8).

## Content With the Contents of Our Plates

Though greed and gluttony promote long-term weight gain, they are not the whole culprit, because gluttony isn't simply overindulgence—it's not being thankful for what we have. Our lack of genuine satisfaction means we don't take the time to see the goodness in the food, so we pile more on our plates than we ever should and gobble things down without even tasting them. This lack of contentment keeps us always wanting more or something different, because in our minds what we have before us isn't good enough.

When summing up the various biblical definitions of the word contentment, it comes down to the idea of being okay with what you have no matter the circumstances. To combat our greedy gluttonous appetites, we need to repent of that sinful notion that makes us think what we have is not quite enough, and then we can learn contentment (Luke 3:14; Phil. 4:11).

The secret to being content isn't changing our portion in life, but finding satisfaction in it. We need to learn to be grateful for what God has given us, no matter what the item or circumstance is. This application works in both eating as well as other life situations. Contentment takes into account God's gracious, all-knowing character and it sees everything as having been put into our lives purposefully. When we aren't content, we forget that God orchestrates all of our events for specific purposes, coupled with His commands for our lives, and we become unhappy and frustrated—and yield to our proclivity to sin.

Only when we genuinely learn to be content with both the right amount and type of food we have on our plates will we begin to take the tiger of our appetites by the tail and be ready to eat repentantly.

We have such an abundance of knowledge on what's nutritionally correct when it comes to proportionate eating—but what we're looking for instead is a magic bullet to take the weight off fast instead of just doing the right thing and letting our bodies reset themselves. So we either severely deny ourselves, or find ways to game the system when we eat with abandon and work out like fiends to burn it off later.

God doesn't condone either of those solutions. He doesn't approve of the "pull the trigger first and say sorry after" mentality that motivates restrictive dieting or excessive exercising (Ps 51:16-17). These things only remove the consequences of the sin but aren't true repentance. Like everything with God, repentant eating is very simple: it just means eating less.

Repentant eating is a meal-by-meal choice if you're someone whose struggle is greed. Not everyone has this magnetic pull toward eating more than we need and may not understand it, but it's important for you to see that since this sin is just like others, we need to battle it just as earnestly. While I don't have to avert my eyes when a hot guy walks by, I do have to avoid an all-you-can-eat buffet on occasion because I know I won't be satisfied with just one trip to the bar. It's a battle I still must wage although the days of being 312 pounds are far behind me. However before I could get to the point where I could say *behind* me, I had to start somewhere. So here is where I started.

# Becoming Your Own Diet Coach

God doesn't leave us without direction and a way to tackle our struggles (1 Cor. 10:13). The problem is, we've heard the directions, but we don't think they apply to us.

So often we believers hear God's good news, except all we hear God say is, "I love you so much I gave up my Son to die in your place and now you're forgiven." And then we don't hear anything else beyond that regarding active repentance. Like that teacher from the Charlie Brown cartoon, all we hear is, "Wah, wah, wa-wa-wa-wahhhhh."

If you're saved, believe it or not, even before you purchased this book, you knew what you needed to produce fruits in keeping with your repentance, regarding your appetite or anything else. Hearkening back to little Zaccheus (Luke 19:1–10), we see that he was the one who came up with the specifics of his repayment plan. Jesus only said, *"hurry and come down, for today I must stay at your house"* (v. 5). While people often need things spelled out for them (Luke 3:7–9), we can find the plan of repentance simply by applying what we've already heard but not heeded.

As He did with Zaccheus, God has asked to come into your house so you too can come up with your plan of repentance in light of being in His presence. You can become your own appetite coach once you move past the "You're saved and forgiven" part of the good news. You are now able to apply the rest of it—that you're saved, forgiven and *you need to live in light of what God's doing in your life.*

You need only cull through the warnings and advice that people have given you along the way to put together the beginnings of a plan, as long as what you've learned doesn't conflict with God's commands. God works through His Word, and He also works through the words of others. However, we may ignore their interventions because we think, in our pride, that the destructions we've been warned against or the remedies offered don't really apply to us. Yet the Bible admonishes us that a person who ignores repeated warnings is going to get their just desserts—and I don't mean the tasty kind either (Prov. 29:1).

Leading up to the time I finally repented, I can think of several times I was reproved to lose weight or advised on how to do it. My father told me I needed to lose the weight before I had a heart attack, my friend Carol who I've mentioned, prayed for me with tears that I would lose weight, while another time her husband gave me practical advice to take fewer tacos at a meal, to name a few instances where God used people in my life. Yet I ignored those warnings and many others I received and became like a fool who pulls the covers back over her head after hearing her house is on fire.

Had I listened, I would have heard, "Repent! Your destruction is certain; cry out to the Lord for help, and eat less."

That changed when I finally crossed the line between being saved to being saved to obey.

# A Simple Plan

As I sat on my bed that day after making the decision to turn my appetite over to God, I thought to myself, profoundly,

*. . . Er . . . now what?*

The "what" came as I decided to apply James 4:17 to come up with a plan to master my appetite.

All of those warnings swirled around my head along with all the bits of helpful advice I'd received over the years. All the times I'd paid to do weight loss programs, or spent money to go to the gym with a trainer or seen the random articles in the doctor's office on nutrition. The Holy Spirit brought everything to mind—so many things that so many people had told me, yet I was doing none of them.

Man's wisdom often works to get you results, but it needs to be weighed against biblical truth. I had to throw out a lot of past ideas I learned about eating if I found they contradicted the idea that Christ said it isn't the food that goes in that defiles us. I took all the warnings and bits of advice and decided to start with those to train my appetite. It was the right thing to do, and I already knew it. I didn't need to learn anything else; I just needed to apply what I had heard.

Okay . . . here goes . . .

- Eat less food.
- Eat a variety of foods.
- Use a smaller spoon.
- Eat three meals and three snacks.
- Drink water.
- Take time to see and appreciate your food.
- Intentionally exercise.

# Eat Less Food

If you're like I was, you lack the ability to govern yourself when it comes to appetite, so you need to agree to a restriction to contain it, even if it feels artificial at first.

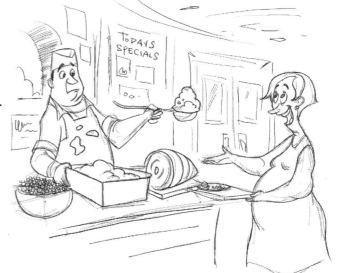

You heard right. I'd like a handful of garlic mashed potatoes please.

When I started this odyssey, I said to Him. "God I got here by being a glutton, so now I'm going to just obey you and use the self-control you've given me. I will let You bring the results. I don't know if I have one day, one week or one year left to live, but whatever life I have left; I want to live it to Your glory."

When I first started changing my eating habits, I ate everything—just less of it. I knew that the biggest issue I had was eating too much, so I had to train myself what was enough. I'd heard that a person should portion their protein the size of their hand. So that's what I started doing, eating the size of my hand not only with protein, but also with the starches/grains and fruits. Vegetables, I ate a little more of, because they're mostly water and could be more satisfying.

For the first year I used the measuring device God had given me: if it fit in my hand I ate it. If the fruit was the size of my fist, that was my serving. If I'd reach into a bag or box of pasta or nuts or whatever, I ate what came out I taught myself to be satisfied with that as my serving.

If I cooked a piece of meat, I would literally hold my hand over it, and anything that extended beyond the side of my palm got cut off. Same for potatoes: If it was outside of my clenched fist, off with its head! When I looked at my plate, none of the portion sizes looked bigger than my palm or fist. As time passed, I started using a scale and measuring cup at home—because it's just too messy to grab a hand full of pasta sauce from the pot.

After a while, my brain got used to seeing smaller portions as enough.

## Eat a Variety of Foods

*Every person is to be in subjection to the governing authorities. For there is no authority except from God, and those which exist are established by God. Therefore whoever resists authority has opposed the ordinance of God; and they who have opposed will receive condemnation upon themselves. For rulers are not a cause of fear for good behavior, but for evil. Do you want to have no fear of authority? Do what is good and you will have praise from the same; for it is a minister of God to you for good. But if you do what is evil, be afraid; for it does not bear the sword for nothing; for it is a minister of God, an avenger who brings wrath on the one who practices evil. Therefore it is necessary to be in subjection, not only because of wrath, but also for conscience' sake.     Rom. 13:1–5*

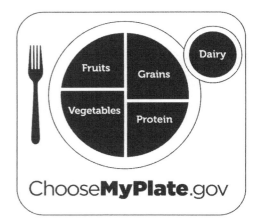

That day as I sat on my bed, my Bible on my lap, asking myself what I should be eating, I knew I had to restrict my intake. But what were the guidelines for what I should chose? I remembered Romans 13:1–5 and then I thought back to my childhood and the food pyramid, a set of guidelines developed by the United States Department of Agriculture designed to help people pick foods that will give them the right nutrition for the needs of the day. With that in mind, I gleefully went to the Internet to refresh my memory as to what I was supposed to eat only to discover—

The food plate had replaced the food pyramid.[19]

So I roughly based my dietary choices on the department of Agriculture's plate info-

---

[19] The MyPlate icon is credited to the U.S. Department of Agriculture (USDA), which does not imply in any way USDA endorsement of this book.

graphic. As I ate within moderation, chose food to suit my tastes and didn't say anything was bad, God gave me so much liberty that eating repentantly became a source of gratitude, not an onerous chore. But lest you think that all I ate was burgers and fries when I first started, let me let you in on a little secret about how I chose what to eat.

Over time, once I'd learned to eat smaller portions, I chose to eat better selections. While, as I said, all food is made by God and neither morally bad or good, however some foods can make us feel either like superslugs or like superheroes. If the issue is to live our lives to be able to love God with all our heart, mind and strength (Luke 10:25–28), then we need to be careful to be moderate in things that hamper the function of our heart, mind and strength.

We all have to eat, but in this world afflicted by sin, our bodies respond differently to different foods. While we need to be careful not to be caught up in the latest nutritional diet fad, we *should* listen to what our body is telling us about what we put into it. It's happier with some choices over others. That's why I think losing weight slowly is actually a blessing even though it's a challenge. The blessing is that you learn what your body can or cannot tolerate. So I'm not saying you can't have pizza . . . I'm just saying weigh how you feel after having that taco pizza against your functionality for the Lord after eating it. If you're curled up in a ball like a fat cat in the sun, then maybe that's not the best choice for you.

Eating experimentally and listening to my body *taught me to see which foods made me feel better*. Not that any of the food I ate was bad, but I saw that some food made me feel light on my feet, while some made me feel as though I'd literally swallowed a stone.

While I'm hesitant to jump on any of those current "eat this, no, no, eat that" food trends, I discovered over time that my body actually didn't like lots of grains or dairy—but it also didn't like corn, white potatoes or white rice either, so I replaced them brown rice, quinoa and sweet potatoes. *But that's just me.*

Likewise, when you find what works for you regarding food, be kind. I've seen so many people become food Nazis when it comes to demanding everyone eat the way that works for them. Stop it.

As I changed my food choices, my tastes eventually changed. I used to go late at night to the greasy burger joint down the street and get a pastrami burger and large fries, but recently I chuckled as I made a late night run to the local grocery store because I was craving sugar snap peas. Yes I have the occasional burger, pizza or taco now and then, but they don't fill me with as much joy as they used to.

Okay, I lied . . . Tacos still make me incredibly happy.

In the end, my food choices are my food choices. If you can eat from the basket of charity bread they set at the table in restaurants and still have a cognitive thought the next day at work, I salute you—I also hate you. Again, it's not what you eat that makes you keep or put on more weight, it's the amount.

## Use a Smaller Spoon

When I spoke about patience in eating, I encouraged you to slow down. I'd heard that eating from a smaller plate tricked your brain into seeing your portion sizes were enough, but since I didn't want to go out and buy new plates I replaced the concept by eating with a smaller spoon. When I did that it actually helped me slow down because I had to take more bites to finish my meal. More bites gave my body more time to realize I was satisfied with the portions I had.

## Eat Three Meals and Three Snacks

I learned from the books I read and the weight loss programs I attended that eating three meals and three snacks throughout the day keeps your metabolism going more effectively. While I can't find that in the Bible, I just do it because I generally do get hungry between meals when I eat normal portions instead of my gargantuan ones.

## Drink Water

Water fills you up and flushes the toxins out of your system. Come on, do I need to say this? We all know this, but we like soda-pop and our coffee drinks better. The result is we gain extra weight from all the sugar in the soda and we can't drink enough coffee to hydrate us. So really, water is the best choice. Water was yick when I first started making it a part of my eating habit, but now I prefer it to anything else.

## Take Time to See and Appreciate Your Food

Having TVs and being able to go out with friends is a fun thing: but if you struggle with gluttony, make sure you take a moment to acknowledge what you have in front of you. I find the times that I don't see my food are the times I struggle later with feeling unsatisfied.

## Intentionally Exercise

I've written a whole chapter on exercise so I wont go into it here, except to say. It needs to be intentional. People are broken into different classifications in terms of activity levels:
- Sedentary
- Moderately active
- Active

I think we can pretty much agree that none of us reading this book are in the "Active" camp.

So we need to incorporate more movement into our lives above what we normally do. Even moms who chase after kids or teachers who stand all day would benefit from making the time to intentionally exercise. Your body gets used to the level of activity you give it. So you need to incorporate more exercise, beyond your normal level of activity. If you're honest with yourself, you eat more food than you need for how active you are, so as I said, you need to spend that food money.

So there you have it . . . the plan I implemented that resulted in my losing weight. The thing I've learned through this whole process is that eating, like exercise, is not one-size-fits-all. Just as you're not sinning if you hate weight lifting, but love going on long walks, you're not sinning if you choose to forgo some foods if they make you feel gross. Just because God made all of them doesn't mean they all work the same for everyone. As long as it's received with thankfulness and contentment from Him who made it, it's ALL good.

The Bible says those who sin do it by practice; they do it over and over until they're masters at it. Through the pages of this book, hopefully you've learned that you're sinning when you're being greedy and so you need to practice eating less while also adding more physical activity, even if it's difficult for a time. While laws can do nothing to restrict the longings of your heart, submitting to them as a trainer will both strengthen your habits of righteousness as well as train you to love from your heart the things God says are good. Once those areas of willful sin are being addressed routinely, your practice of them will become a happy habit and not a robot action.

After about a year of slow and steady weight loss I ran into a mom from my church in a local store. She was a bit overweight, so she asked me how I was losing mine. I mentioned the concept of applying James 4:17 to avoiding the wrong I knew to be true. She said thoughtfully as we stood there in the crackers and cookies aisle next to a giant shelf loaded with cheesy snack crackers, "I learned that I should shop the periphery of the store for healthy choices." I'd never heard that before, but I smiled because I was doing that since I'd changed my eating. I barely visited the middle of the store anymore unless I was baking someone cookies. I then went on to encourage her with the words "Since you know that, then you should stay out of aisles like these."

**Take a moment to write down all the things you know are the right things to do for you in order to come up with your own plan to practice righteousness in the area of obedient eating.**

# When Your Tongue Literally Gives You Reason to Praise

The first lesson I learned when I lost weight while eating fewer french fries was that food was not the awful scoundrel I'd made it to be: its only purpose was to help me live.

For those of you who have *actual* health issues regarding food—please don't think I'm telling you to go out and eat something that's clearly going to do you harm. I'M NOT A DOCTOR as I said before. Don't take any medical advice from a cartoonist.

My admonition to take food from the naughty list is for those who *can* eat anything but think the problem lies in the choices of their food, so they go on a diet. Diets become problematic because not only does it wrongly place the blame on something outside of you, it also shuts off an avenue to praise God.

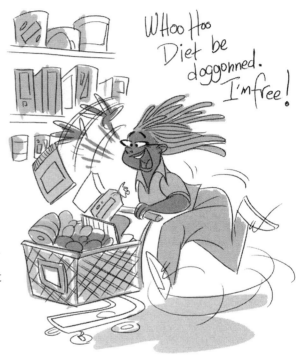

God's great gift in food is not the food itself, but rather that the food is a larger part of His creative design. He has given us taste buds to enjoy our food, and then He made food to stimulate those taste buds, all to make sure His little creatures would remember to eat through the day. So instead of booting this food or that, give thanks to Him for making food taste, oh, so good. After all, you *could* be eating vitamin-fortified cardboard.

How twisted would it be for the Creator to make those two things, taste buds and food—but then say, "Hah, but you can only eat _____?" God is not a sadistic tyrant sitting on His throne in heaven with a giant whacker to swat your hand when you reach for a cookie!

Let me insert here that Jesus said if something causes you to stumble, then you need to cut it off completely (Matt. 18:8–9). So if you have certain foods that you refuse to have control over, then you aren't in the wrong to avoid them like the plague.

As I ate anything I wanted within reason, I found myself not only losing weight, but also being incredibly thankful to God who created those foods and gave them to me as gifts. All I'm encouraging you to consider is the portion sizes over the portion choices. The thing about gifts is that no matter how good they are, they can turn into clutter if you have too many of them. Too much food gifts makes FAT clutter.

Most diets these days attack the gift of food, and while it works to take off the weight, it only works for so long. Eventually the handcuffs of dieting makes you and I want to give up completely or at least make bargains with ourselves like:

"Well I was great for lunch today; I can have a little more for dinner."

. . . or . . .

"My diet says I can have all I want of (fill in the blank) and still lose weight!"

When I focused on the amount of food instead of the type of food, I was able to quit beating myself up over it and rejoice about a small piece of carrot cake or a single barbeque rib I had at the party. Of course as we learn to eat what suits our body functions we see there are definitely better choices than others but that doesn't exempt us from the notion of seeing what we have on our plate with gratitude and for its right purpose. Otherwise, we can be just as sinfully greedy while eating sweet peppers as we can eating pepperoni pizza.

## The Right Reason to Party

It's a lot easier to control your food when you're at home, but so much of our interaction with others is around food. So what do we do about parties and family gatherings? It's easy in situations like these to become a Food Pharisee.

The Pharisees were hypocritical religious people living during the time of Jesus who practiced their brand of religion but had no real devotion to God. Oftentimes they justified their abuse and neglect of the people they should have been serving by cloaking their actions in their warped, self-serving application of religion (Matt. 23:23–28). When Jesus went toe-to-toe with them, the Pharisees responded like the petulant children that they were, lobbing back the insult, "Oh, yeah, well you fatso drunk" because they saw Jesus routinely attended dinner parties in the course of His ministry (Luke 7:34).

In the example of these two parties, Jesus and the Pharisees, we can find a lesson for how we should face our holidays and dinner parties. While the Pharisees went to large social gatherings to be seen, Jesus went to dinner parties *because of the people He wanted to see* (Matt. 23:6–7; Matt. 9:11–13).

The most important thing to remember in our striving to be like Christ in situations like this is not only the command to be controlled, but also the exhortation to be compassionate. We need to interact with the people we love and who love us enough to cook us meals, so we can discern their needs and serve or pray for them. Of course there'll be food at those events so we need to be vigilant and apply all the things we've learned through the pages of this book—to take what we want and walk away, to avoid the things that may cause us to stumble, to eat slowly and gratefully—but above all we need to focus more on the partygoers than the party platters.

There's a time for feasting and there's a time to abstain, but when there's a time for eating, let us be like Christ who ate all the food placed before Him with gratitude until he was satisfied or maybe even missed the meal because He was so engrossed in doing His

Father's work regarding the needs of the person in front of Him (John 4:32) instead of being like the Pharisees who for all their right actions still grumbled against Jesus Christ, God incarnate, who was trying to turn them from their path of destruction.

# Weaving It All Together

Earlier in the chapter I wrote briefly about the topic of contentment in regard to eating in response to our circumstances, but I would like to address it a bit more here. In the end, we need to eat for the sake of sustaining the machine, instead of for any of the other reasons we commonly eat, even the emotional ones. God sees us in our times of despair, fear, and brokenheartedness, and He knows that the only lasting satisfaction is found in Him, not in all the things that we turn to instead (Pss. 6:8–9; 42; 56; 116:1–9). We need to turn to God and resist the urge to control our lives when we don't like our situations and food seems to be the only way to do it. We need to remember we can only see just so much of what our lives have in store for us.

Years ago a friend a mine had the privilege of executing the artwork in the castle at an amusement park in Paris. He was responsible for all the character art which meant he designed and oversaw the stained glass windows, the faux story books and several large tapestries . . . and they spared no expense. The windows were done in England by somebody who serves the royal family, the books were done stateside, and the elaborate loomed tapestries, valued at multiple thousands of dollars, were done at an establishment in Brussels. It was a glorious display when it was put together. A few years after it opened, I went to see the "attraction," and as I patiently filed around the room packed with eager viewers, I saw a man reach across the velvet rope toward an intricate tapestry. The park-goer clutched the edge of the delicate, colorful piece and flipped it up, wanting to see if it was indeed a real tapestry or basically a glorified towel. "Ne touche pas!" I hissed *sotto voce,* "Don't touch it. It's art!" the man, startled, immediately released his grasp of the tapestry with a meek "pardon," and hurried on his way. He'd only wanted to see the handiwork, the artful hideous knots that proved the art was the real deal and not a counterfeit.

God's children are the real deal and our lives are His art. We have to take it on faith that our life tapestry is a beautiful one, because we can only see the backside with its knotty bits.

It's the knots behind the tapestry, artfully done, that brought my friend's creation to a beautiful representation . . . and yet, when we encounter tangles and knots in our own lives, we think "Ugh, this is ugly. How's this ever going to work out? And since I can't untie this knot, how can I make myself happy in it?"

When God places us in situations that are seemingly knotty and tangled, how can we address our frustrated desires in a practical way that doesn't involve eating?

Consider the character of the Artist of your life. He is so much greater than my extremely talented friend who art-directed a castle for a multi-billion dollar company. God knows just how to make things beautiful in their appointed time (Eccl. 3:11). This returns to our encouragement to grow in the knowledge of who God is: asking Him to open the eyes of our heart to see Him more clearly while we continue to do what we know to be right even though our hearts are aching.

No, I don't do this perfectly all the time. I have seasons of successfully staying in the midst of the knots and other times when I treat my trials like a game of "cat's cradle" and try and change the knots into something else. God knows His planned design, so all of my reworking, controlling and scheming aren't going to change it. So I have to remind myself not try to control it by means of schemes or try to make myself happy by overeating.

Ultimately, when I want to eat something beyond being hungry (if I'm not being just plain old greedy), it's be-cause I am not satisfied where God is taking me in my life. To be discontented with the situation I'm in is to say, in essence, "God, I don't think You know what You're doing. You're not making art, but a garbage heap of my life. Can't you see I'm suffering here?"

God is completely sovereign over all that happens in our lives. So when pain comes, we need to pour out our concerns to the Lord but also change our attitudes toward the events He has orchestrated. Like a guitar string that has gotten slightly flat, we need to tune ourselves against what's true about God as revealed in His Word regarding our

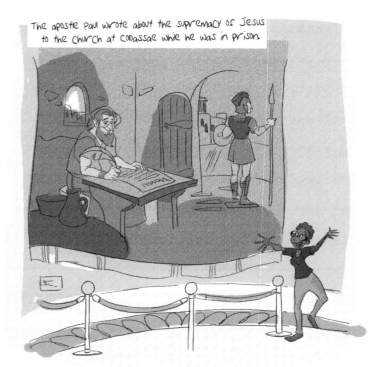

The apostle Paul wrote about the supremacy of Jesus to the church at Colassae while he was in prison.

*Are you making the most of your knotty circumstances?*

situation and His character. Then we choose to yield our hearts to accept what He's orches-trated as part of His perfect plan.

Ugh. It may not feel perfect to me at the time, but it is perfect in light of the fact that He can see everything down the road.

God knows the design for the art of our lives. So we obey what we know to be true instead of running to our sin, because God who sees down the road has a purpose yet to be revealed (1 Pet. 1:3–9).

That being said, if you and I tried to live obediently for "down the road," we'd give up in frustration because it's too difficult to think that far beyond the horizon. God doesn't want us to live for down the road—He'll take care of that. Instead, He wants us to trust Him today—right now—moment by moment. I used to say to a group of high school kids I worked with, "I don't know what could happen tomorrow, I could get hit by a semi truck." To which one of them eventually replied, "I wish you'd stop saying that; it makes me uncomfortable."

One day I *was* hit by a semi, and you know what? God spared my life!

The point is, we don't know our futures. God wants us to trust Him right now in whatever painful, boring, or lonely situation He orchestrates in our lives. We need to resist the temptation to find comfort in our greed. He wants us not to run from Him in trials, but to *rest* in Him in our trial.

You could say it would be a lot easier if food tasted meh, because then you wouldn't be a glutton. But no, the problem of your disobedient heart would be there whether or not it was fueled by a Philly cheesesteak with a side of fries and some of your friend's fries to boot. Trust me, I've been in places where the food was terrible and still I was a piggie. No the problem isn't that food tastes good; it's that we worship the creation and how it makes us feel instead of the God who created it.

Though it's challenging to slay my appetite, the more I do it—halting, stumbling, but always getting up looking to my Father—the farther I make it before I stumble again. I think, *God, I'm lonely, or bored or angry, but it's You who has ordained that I be single or home-bound or allowed me to lose my job, or had someone bring an amazing banana cream pie to this potluck* [all hypothetical—except for the pie] *and since You're perfect, help me to trust that this moment in time that's making me upset, lonesome, covetous, or bored is Yours.* And then . . . *I make the choice not to eat.*

It's not that I'm suddenly, *Zow, I feel amazing and now that extra Pizza isn't an option.* No, it's, *I still feel pretty lousy and I still want the pizza, but I value the relationship with God more than the option to sin, and I know that if I choose to sin, I break the relationship. . . . So I'd rather suffer this bored, lonely, frustrated circumstance, because having communion with Him is so much sweeter.*

Eventually God changes my heart to be content in the painful, bored, lonely or frustrating circumstance . . . but sometimes it takes a while to get to the point where I can say, "It is well with my soul." In those times I'm thankful I have friends who are fellow believers who can pray with me and talk me off the ledge when my trials are too much for me to bear by faith alone.

In the end, that's how weight loss by repentant eating is not solely the goal-oriented "When I lose 161 pounds, then I stop" kind of thing. No it's a life change, because our attitude toward food should remain the same even after the weight comes off—otherwise it will eventually creeeeep . . . back . . . on.

Repentant eating is about moderately eating and being thankful for what's in front of you, whether its a kale salad or a bit of a grill cheese dipper with tomato soup. Having a bunch of rules is a lot easier to follow, because then it feels like you're doing it right—but in the end, rules don't really change you from the inside and after a while you start to rebel against them if you don't address the real problem: your sinful heart. If you go on a diet you just lose the weight. If you repentantly eat you learn patience, gratitude, contentment, self-control and faithfulness. You gain eyes to see your heavenly Father who loves you— *and you lose the weight too!*

Christians live to love God and love their neighbors as themselves. The chief end of repentant eating is to be ready both physically and with our attitudes to serve one another. If we're only doing it to look good, then we're only aiming at the tiniest non-important aspect of our existence. We weren't made to be worshiped—only God deserves that—but as we strive to glorify God with our lives we can love and be loved. We were made to give comfort to others and can receive comfort from others as well. As we cultivate godly hearts as a replacement for our sinful ones we grow in our ability to offer the comfort, service and love others need, and if we're hurting, we also have the humility to receive it from others, as well. In the remaining chapters of this book I'll discuss the goal of repentant eating: to equip us to obey God's call to love one another as ourselves.

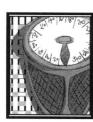 # Take A-Weigh

- To change your eating habits, just start being faithful in what you already know what to do.
- People are the point of parties, not the food.
- God hasn't forgotten you in your trials. Don't turn to another god to comfort yourself.

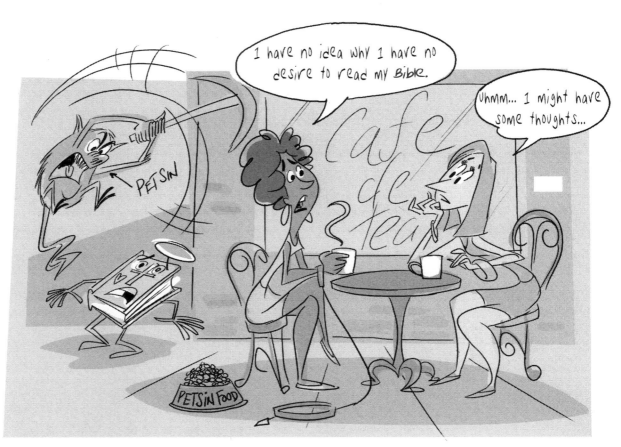

We don't have to do this walk alone.

Chapter 14

# Tearing Down the Kingdom of Me

I was sitting by the side of the road shivering with fear and near tears. Three miles . . . *three lousy miles* stood between me and the Chantry parking lot! Three miles—and a windy mountain road.

There's a series of peaks nicknamed the Six Pack; each one progressively taller than the last. Hikers climb them so that they can ready themselves to tackle Mount Whitney. I'd asked three other ladies to join me one Saturday morning for the six-hour, fifteen-mile out and back 5712-foot Mount Wilson hike just outside of Pasadena, California, and I had gone to scout the location the day before we went.

It never occurred to me that hiking on a mountain would first mean driving on one! I was so terrified as I slowly drove along the well-maintained but cliffside mountain road, that I eventually turned back before I reached the trailhead.

I was flummoxed and embarrassed; here I was, the leader of an event, but I was too weak to lead because of my fear. How was I going to ever get Whitney's pinnacle if I couldn't even get to Wilson's parking lot now?

I prayed to God for a solution and, though I was embarrassed, I texted one of the other hikers and explained my situation.

"So I just tried to drive up to the parking and I'm wondering would you mind driving my car tomorrow or can one of the other ladies drive their car up there? It's a narrow two-lane road that is 3 miles long but I can't do it especially in the dark because of my fear of heights... And with four women yammering in the car I'll be even more terrified :( sorry I didn't realize that parking would be so far up!"

My friend's immediate and nonjudgmental response was, "Sure, no problem."

When faced with the mountains God calls us to obediently summit, we can find ourselves in a struggle to tackle what might appear to others around us as a simple command. In a world that screams louder than God's gentle whisper, our flesh is too weak, our ears too deaf and our hearts to faint at times to access God's gifts to lead us home. We can be incapacitated by our emotions, hamstrung by our own laziness and reluctant to let go of the sin that makes us happy, all the while ardently desiring to be *set free from those very things!*

God has compassion for the weakness of His feeble little creatures. One way He provides the answer to our struggle to obey Him is in the application of the royal law to love God and love our neighbors as ourselves. We first need to turn to God in prayer for help but we need to rely on one another for guidance as well. It's in seeking our brothers and sisters in the body of Christ that we can find support when we're weak, encouragement when we're down-hearted, exhortation when we're lazy, and edification when we're misinformed. But we must be willing to venture out from own little kingdoms of self-preservation to find the help we so desperately need.

## While You're Not Alone, You're All You Have

When Jesus met with His disciples in the last hours before His death, not only did He promise them a helper in the Holy Spirit, He reminded them they needed to watch out for one another. The world hates Jesus and everyone associated with His message. So it will do everything in its power, from killing professing believers to tempting them to surrender to their weakness, in order to stop the spread of the gospel of God's merciful salvation. Even the nicest nonbeliever friend will at one point try to stop a Christian from glorifying God in their fight against sin with a sweet, "Don't be so hard on yourself, you're only human . . . " when what the Christian needs to hear is, "God died for that sin; yes, you've fallen in your weak humanity and I'm sorry for what you're going through so I'll be praying for you, but *get up and keep going to His glory!"*

So Jesus told His disciples to love one another, and two thousand years later the command remains the same for us. We're to show that love for one another by meeting each other's needs as God gives us the resources, whether it's physical needs or manual service or the more emotional and spiritual needs of comfort and guidance.

You aren't alone!

That should thrill your heart to read those words in the battle against your greed. God commands us to be there for one another. By sharing our sins, struggles, and disappointments with each other, not only do we obtain the benefit of their prayers, but we also find accountability.

It seems like a simple thing to say that we need to go to one another for help and accountability but oftentimes it's the last thing we seek because of our pride and the residual affects of our sin.

There are some sins that are so entrenched in our lives that we don't realize how much they separate us from others. We may believe we are open and inviting, but we are blinded to the fact that the attitudes that allow that sin to flourish in our lives are also pushing many others away from us.

After God opens our eyes to the "stinkin' thinkin'" that goes on in our hearts when we sin, we struggle with the belief that if we share our failings, then people will reject us for our ugliness. While some immature and shallow people may shun you for expressing your struggles, you'll find more people who are willing to embrace and encourage you because of them, because even the most "perfect person" you admire in your church is aware of being a grubby little sinner *just like you!* Therefore we need to turn to one another to help us as we apply God's commands to repent and obey.

# Wise Old Words From a Long-Dead Dude

A couple thousand years ago, the preacher in Ecclesiastes wrote about the importance of not living a solitary life (Eccl. 4:9–12). While it may seem simplistic to be reminded that we need to help one another, how many times do you and I just try to do things on our own? As a result, things take longer, aren't done as well or maybe don't even get done at all, because we're just too weak to accomplish the task.

So indulge me while I expound on the ancient words with potential applications for our Christian walk, so that maybe the next time you waffle between reaching out to someone else or not, you'll choose to ask for help rather than go it alone.

*1. You get more return on your work by working with a partner.* "Many hands make light work," so the saying goes. A group of people can get more accomplished than just one person working alone. This applies to everything from cleaning up the tables after a church potluck to reaching out to the widows and single moms in your congregation. For those of you who struggle to get out the door to exercise, you'll find you get more work from your workout when you ask someone to go with you.

*2. You've got someone to pick you up when you fall.* Apart from the obvious application that there's someone to pick you up when your fall physically, you and I need one another to help us when we fall emotionally as well. Who doesn't appreciate encouragement when we need comfort or someone to make us laugh at ourselves when we're taking things too seriously?

Just as a baby needs to know that a stumble is not the end of the world, we too need to see that each time we fall, it isn't the end of the story; it's just a temporary owie. That's why we need people to pick us up, dust us off or help us heal, before they send us on our way. Woe to the person who falls alone: they can be broken both physically as well as emotionally.

When we're working to overcome our sin there are going to be times when we run like the wind, but there'll also be times when we stumble and fall. The people closest to us, with their prayers, encouragement and advice, won't let us stay down too long.

*3. You can stay warm when it's cold.* While in the days of Solomon when there was no central heating, the concept of warmth was more a practical one. In our current time, the concept of warmth becomes an emotional or spiritual one. How often we find that when our emotions or faith has grown cold that being in the presence of someone who's on fire for God can melt the frost that makes our hearts brittle.

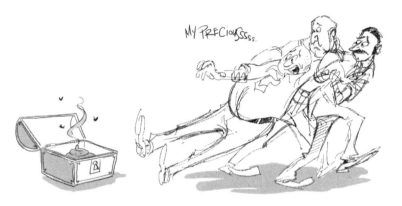

MY PRECIOUSSSSS.

But encourage one another day after day, as long as it is still called "Today," so that none of you will be hardened by the deceitfulness of sin. Heb 3:13

This is different from being picked up after we've stumbled, because stumbling implies motion toward something before falling, whereas growing cold indicates we've either stopped or walked away from the source of heat. It's a foolish person who thinks they can go this hard, hard life alone, away from others who share God's calling, for when that solitary person loses the passion of their first decision they lose also their focus and direction. We need to surround ourselves with people who can stoke the fire in our walk when our repentance grows cold.

*4. You gain a source of protection when someone attacks you.* The world isn't as dangerous as it was in Solomon's age when kingdoms went to war against each other and carried away captives at the drop of a helmet—*or is it?* There are people in countries outside of the United States that are literally being thrown in jail or slaughtered for their faith. Even without the threat of a jihad, Christians can have enemies. The apostle Paul said that those who desired to live righteously would face persecution (2 Tim. 3:12). That's why we need to watch each other's backs with prayer or physically stand with one another in the face of attack. While sometimes a united front will deter our enemies, other times, even though we may suffer loss, we can find comfort in knowing we have people standing with us. As the saying goes, "Grief shared is half grief; joy shared is double joy."

There are times when we need to provide and receive protection in the church as well. Sometimes our old nature makes us targets for distrust; look at Paul after his conversion (Acts 9:13–15). While no one is going to distrust you for being obese, there might be a lot of attitudes you held in while you were deceived by your sin that now cause people to lift an eyebrow to you as you strive to repentantly incorporate yourself into the body of Christ. In such situations, you need someone who's willing to defend you, even if it's from friendly fire.

*5. You find strength in the company of others.* Single strands of rope have only just so much strength, but together they become formidable. Even as we aren't afraid to admit our weakness to ourselves and to each other, we don't stop there, otherwise we wallow in self-pity. From there we need to come together to encourage and pray for one another, offering one another exhortations from the Bible so that together we become stronger. People who don't admit their spiritual and emotional weakness will eventually snap under the pressures of life, striving to master their sinful desires alone.

Overcoming sin is hard, hard work, because, though God empowers us, we still have to put one foot in front of the other in order to obey Him. We need others in our lives who are authentic in their own vulnerability yet who may also possess spiritual insights so that together we both can advance down the Kingdom road. Actively seek to find others who are stronger than you are, to encourage, pray for and guide you while you seek to follow God's commands to repent.

# Spiritual Walking Buddies

Even if you must start your journey of repentance and obedience alone, you'll eventually find your accountability partner. You might meet with this person weekly for a predetermined length of time or on a long-term basis. In this age of technology, there isn't any reason you can't do it via the phone, video conferencing or social media. Your accountability partner (or group) doesn't necessarily have to share your same struggle with greed, they only have to know and love the Lord, and know how to fight sin in their own lives.

This is more than a free therapy session; it's an opportunity to crack open your Bibles and wrestle with how to apply its truths to your lives in a mutual way. As you're open with each other, you can pray for each other. The person who becomes your accountability partner needs to be patient with you, but you also need to be patient with that person, who is not God, after all, but a fallible human being like you.

Above all, be humble enough to accept the person's input, committed to staying under his or her guidance and encouragement even when it's difficult. It's not going to help you in the long run if you walk away in anger when your accountability partner points out some truth you don't want to hear.

The common factor in finding accountability is humbling yourself to be encouraged by others to follow through on what you've planned, whether they check back with you to make sure you memorized the Bible verses you promised you would master by the following week, or pray for you about a besetting sin and to check back with you from time to time to see how goes the battle, or let you text them at night with something you learned in your Bible reading for the day.

While these few elements of accountability can be done somewhat casually and in small groups, all of these aspects of accountability can fit quite nicely into the big show: personal discipleship.

## Some Assembly Required

If you look at Jesus with His disciples you'll see what a discipleship relationship looks like. The apostles spent intense time with the Lord learning about the Kingdom of heaven from Him, getting their rough edges sanded down, finding out how they were supposed to behave as believers and seeing how Jesus related to the people outside of their inner circle. We need to prayerfully seek to cultivate this kind of relationship with those who are stronger than us, as we seek to battle the sin in our lives and grow as believers.

In this form of accountability, you seek someone who's spiritually stronger than you and you commit to be under his or her mentorship for a time. Mentors let you into their lives so you can learn by example as they navigate in their world. They speak the truth of God's Word into your life, even when it's hard to hear at the time. They'll also pray for you and show you compassion.

How do you find this person? For me, it was while I was trying to be that type of person to someone who was spiritually more needy than I was. Some of the most edifying relationships I've found have been when I've been serving other people, not when I've been looking for someone to serve me. When we focus less on ourselves, we're open to see the great things in other people that we wish we had. Think of it as a mini reward for obeying the Jesus command to make disciples. If we're doing our part to fulfill Christ's great commission, even in our weakened state, we'll eventually come under the tutelage of someone who sees where we could grow; we will find others from whom we can learn.

I met Robin while I was a youth leader to her daughter in our church high school group. Over the years Robin did all of those things in my life that Jesus did with His disciples. I met with her weekly and her life was an open book. She was endlessly patient, and was committed to me for many years of my minimal change and knuckleheaded stubbornness. Over the years I saw her in wonderful times with her family, and also in difficult trials of her husband's illness. Not only did she hang in there with me until I was finally able to break the back of several of my connected besetting sins, she also taught me through the way she faced her trials the lesson that God is good all the time, even when we struggle. In the end, though I went to her to help me overcome a specific sin, Robin helped me grow in my relationship to Christ as well as understand my role as a woman in the church. A good discipleship relationship is like that, we are like pancakes, not waffles, when it comes to the outpouring of God's sweet transforming grace—His work isn't just going to stay in one pocket of your life; it's going to get all over you.

Discipleship relationships aren't very successful if you don't put in the work yourself; you actually need to do something with the counsel your discipler gives you, even if it's only to say, "Help me understand how to make your advice work in my life . . . " You should be able to go to your discipler with your questions about what you hear in church, what you read in the Bible, or how to apply God's commands to your life.

While disciplers help you implement God's commands, they don't know your heart like you do: so you need to tell them where you want to grow to start the process. You need to set up with them what your goals are and what you want to work on and they can help you get there with their spiritual experience. Eventually over time you might both discover that the issue that presented itself for fixing was only the flower of a bigger, more gnarly, plant underneath—but you won't find out if you don't start with a desire to obey God and change in mind. I didn't go to Robin to deal with my greed, but instead something else. However, when God finally changed my heart regarding my appetite, she rejoiced with me. During that summer of change, she'd walk with me on the cool Thursday evenings when we met for our times of discipleship. The investment of her years of encouragement and exhortation spurred me on to battle my sin of greed but the marvelous thing was because God removed the issue of greed, I was then able to finally hear her sharp rebuke to repent of the other area I had come to her for help with in the first place. She was a spiritual leader who eventually became a spiritual running mate.

## Care and Feeding of Your Soul's Caretaker

The Bible teaches that those who help others in need should discern the level of their interaction: An unruly person should be admonished, a fainthearted person should be encouraged and a weak person should be helped, but all of them should receive patience (1 Thess. 5:14). Are you unruly, fainthearted or weak? We need to check our hearts to see where we fall on that list when we're coming under someone for accountability.

You're what the Bible labels as unruly if your life and attitude is characterized by being disorderly, irregular, inordinate, or immoderate, and you find yourself routinely deviating from the prescribed order or rule. If your life shows discouragement then you're fainthearted; if you're infirm and feeble, then you're weak. You may be weak because you're physically sick or because you've been emotionally abused. You may be fainthearted because you've tried in the past to battle your sin but have fallen back into old patterns. Or you may very well be unruly because you're either stubborn or simply too lazy to try at all. You know your heart. You have to be honest with yourself and start from there.

To those of you who may realize you're unruly, understand that your discipler isn't a miracle-worker; he or she is a human being just like you. You must put in the work of applying what they recommend, making certain you're not making your discipler's job harder by how we apply their counsel. While God gives people wisdom and patience through the trials in their lives, you don't want to be a source of more trials that force your discipler to ask for God's wisdom to bear with you!

I know transformation at times is difficult, but get out of that whole unruly thing as quickly as you can. Seek the Lord through prayer and reading His Word. Apply the counsel of your discipler. Understand that it's you who has the problem when you're bunching up your back at God's commands. Consider the love of God who gave up His Son to save your life and beg His forgiveness and ask Him to help you change your contentious spirit.

No matter where you are regarding working with your discipler to tame your gluttonous heart or any pet sin, your goal needs to be the same: to please God with your actions, regardless of the external results.

Bear in mind also: While you meet with an accountability person, don't become so myopic that you shut out other avenues of getting help through all available outlets God provides, such as the following:

*1. Get involved in a Bible study.* Avail yourself of the wisdom that can be gained by joining a group of likeminded believers who sit under a common teacher, and take encouragement from the community there. Corporate Bible studies are excellent places not only to learn what the Bible teaches, but also to encourage one another. Because of your classmates, you can see that you're not alone in your struggles. Accountability is accountability even if it's not intensely one-on-one; start with what you do have.

2. *Be in church as much as you can.* Not because you're trying to prove you're a Christian, but because being in the church gives you an opportunity to learn to love others who are different (Prov. 27:17). As you learn about the buttons people push on you, guess what—you discover other areas where you need to become accountable. Yay?

3. *Don't be afraid to ask questions.* Don't query out of combativeness, but because you seek to understand God, His ways and how He wants you to grow in Him (Prov. 9:7–10; John 6:44–45; Rom. 16:17–18; Eph. 5:8–10; 2 Tim. 3:10–16). If you come with a humble, teachable heart then people will be willing to help.

Jesus said that anyone who comes to Him should come like a child (Mark 10:15). While I believe this means we're to come to Him with the trust of a child, I'd like to apply it also to the idea that everything is new information to children. Their little brains are like sponges soaking up the world. They don't have a sense that everyone else knows the answer to the reason why the sky is blue, so they're not ashamed to ask the question. Don't be afraid to ask your questions about God and His Word, even if you think it's been asked before. Let me encourage you—it already has been. *Lots of times* (and sometimes to the same person). But that doesn't mean you shouldn't ask the question for yourself; that's how you grow.

Do we hold back from walking down a sidewalk because we see our neighbor there first? If our destination is at the end of the block and that's the only way to get there, we go without shame because our goal is in sight. God doesn't condemn our finite minds for not understanding everything about infinite things. It's okay to question the things we don't understand if we're seeking to grow in Him (James 1:5).

4. *Be transparent.* There's that closet in the back room—you know, the one that's got stuff in it no one should see, right? Poppycock. Air that junk! It's impossible to be true kingdom of self-demolishers while keeping things hidden. We hide our deepest fears and struggles: yet we're called to pray for one another. How can we do that if we aren't being transparent while asking for prayer? (James 5:16).

While there's wisdom in not broadcasting the deepest secrets of your heart to every Tammy, Dot and Harriet, we do need to go out on a limb with the trustworthy people in our lives. We need to stop shallowly sharing the most sanitized parts of our lives like someone skipping a stone across a lake, and sometimes just let the big rocks drop with a splash for those trusted few to see.

If we're going to be accountable to people, we actually need to give them something which to hold us accountable.

Once we've shared those dark and secret things with them, we also need to reciprocate and be a safe place for them to turn.

Above all, be careful not to fall into the trap of basing your acceptability on your acceptability to your group (meaning that if you do well they'll be pleased; if you mess up, they'll be disappointed). Focusing on your accountability partner as your measure of righteousness will always give you an out: "Oh, they're human and nobody is perfect; they'll give me a pass." If you are squishy in your repentance, you'll wonder why you haven't been able to find lasting victory over your sin. Remember, these people are only God's servants. The moment you grasp how damaging your sin is to Him, is when your sin will begin to lose its grip on you.

# When Saying "I Love You" Means Saying Hard Things

> *Let us hold fast the confession of our hope without wavering, for He who promised is faithful; and let us consider how to stimulate one another to love and good deeds, not forsaking our own assembling together, as is the habit of some, but encouraging one another; and all the more as you see the day drawing near.* Heb. 10:23–25

The idea is that we're all in this together, even if at times it's as awkward as being in a three-legged race. God calls us to be both contestant and cheerleader, participant and encourager. Nobody wins if we don't win together. Is this some form of Christian communism? No, it's family.

We need to encourage one another to love and good deeds even if at times it's challenging, embarrassing and maybe not even received too well. These next few words are written to those of you who have people in your life who you see are struggling in the area of greed and gluttony. They may come to you for help or they may not, but either way you need to be ready to encourage them in any way you can.

You are so important . . .

You may not be popular with the people in your life who are sinfully eating. You may be ignored. You may be thought of as ungracious or judgmental. But let your love for the greedy people in your life coax you past your fear of rejection. Now I'm not saying walk up to your friend, wife, sister, brother, mother, father, grandma or other and say "Uhm, your bottom's looking rather squishy these days, you might want to lay off a cream puff or twenty." No. Pray for them. I mean it. Really, pray for them. Consider how to encourage them in small ways keeping in mind that maybe the greed is just the tip of the iceberg of some other sin God wants to address first. No matter what, tell them the truth in love (Eph. 4:15–16; Gal. 6:1).

If they ignore you, try not to take it too hard and keep praying. The thing about sin is that those people you love can become hardened by its deceitfulness (Heb. 3:12–13).

Once again, I state for the record that being obese is not the sin, but the idolatry, greed and gluttony that contribute to their long-term weight gain is. Those people entangled in the clutches of greed may have become so inured to the poison bubbling up in their soul that they might need someone to take them by the hand and gently lead them to the mirror of God's grace shown through the pages of the Bible so that they can compare themselves to what they see there instead of what they see with their sin-blinded eyes.

Do this humbly. You may not struggle as your loved one does in the area of food overindulgence, but you too struggle with some powerful sin in another area. No one is perfect, except for Jesus, so while we're called to encourage one another to good deeds it's with the humility of someone who knows they too need encouragement in other areas. So with lowly hearts we guide one another in the areas where each of us is blind, to live in the image of the righteousness of Christ.

Bear in mind two things in your admonition: Make sure you're committed to the person you seek to encourage in an ongoing relationship, because battling with overindulgence is a long-term proposition. If you're going to bring up the issue, let them know you're going to be by their side to walk with them through it. Also, be careful you're not basing your admonishment solely on looks. You don't want to walk up to a freshly minted mommy carrying a diaper bag, a brand-new baby and forty extra pounds of weight

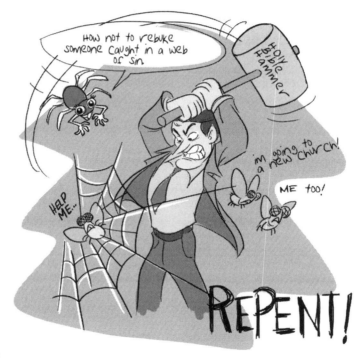

to tell her you want to help them unlock the cause to her obesity, but feel free to broach the subject with a mother of a six-year-old who's still eating for two: remember it's the actions and attitudes, not the appearance, that God addresses. Who knows, you might find you need to confront the sin of greed in your rail-thin friend.

For those of you who struggle with greed and have friends who've gathered their courage to admonish you, compelled by Christ's love overflowing within them—receive their timid admonition with grace. Get over your embarrassment and act on their words even though they're halting, clunky and just difficult to hear. Understand it's not easy to humbly rebuke a brother or sister in their sin. Take their words as your charge to repent.

Obesity is a touchy subject. The reason people don't want to say anything about a person's weight gain is the same reason they don't say anything when you've lost the weight, until it's significant: They don't want to be offensive. However, if we viewed long-term weight gain as matter of sin like adultery or lying, we'd be more likely to confront one another in the love of Jesus, with the same urgency as if we had caught a fellow believer in an illicit affair.

When someone comes to you with the desire to help you, realize it's for your good and because they love you. When people care enough to utter the words, "You have a problem," it's as if they're offering you a precious gift.

## Long-Distance Running

While this is a chapter on accountability, sometimes people who love you enough to say something don't have the time to do anything more than check in on you periodically to see if you're still plugging away at it. While it would have been nice if in those early days someone would have run with me or even walked, the point I want to bring up is that though we're called to encourage one another in our sin struggles, we who seek to obey God in the area of our appetites still need to do the work on our own when we're alone (Gal. 6:5).

The prodigal son did a very good job spending his money when he was living wildly and there were plenty of people to help him do it (Luke 15:11–32), yet when he needed to repent, he willingly changed his ways all alone.

Too many people resist starting this journey (or any siege against their pet sin) because they're overwhelmed by the thought they have to do it without support. We like to sin in private, but repent with a cheering section. Why is this? I think in both cases it's so we can indulge our flesh. While the first one is an obvious reason: if someone sees us sinning then we might have to stop, the other one is not so obvious. It's the excuse "Well, no one is helping me so I guess I don't have to start."

Let me encourage you with this thought: We have the benefit of knowing the end of the prodigal's story, when the father was waiting for him to return. We should set out on this road of repentance whether or not we have accountability in the church, because we know God is waiting for us.

I know how difficult it is to repent in the area of controlling your appetite when you're mostly alone because in the early days, when I first realized what repentant eating was, that's how I did it. I lived alone, so I had to restrict my food while no one was watching, and I exercised alone in all types of weather. I bore the sorrows I would have normally buried in food to the throne of grace. But I was so alone in this battle; I longed for others to join me in my trudge. I understand how hellishly gut-wrenching and painful it is when you're faced with standing on your own two feet *away* from people who can prop you up with a reassuring word and arm around the shoulder. How our bodies wail out for MORE!

Let me encourage you: Even though your flesh whines and weeps, gnashes and yawls, it does it now because you won't have to do it for eternity in hell. The agony you endure while crucifying your appetite on earth is as bad as it ever gets (Rom. 8:18–25).

God has saved us from our soul's despair for eternity in exchange for our killing our sinful desires for our earthly lifetimes (Rom. 8:12–18). When we crucify our flesh we become like Jesus when He died physically. We, along with the ones in our lives who are doing the same, need to pick up our cross with our appetites nailed to it and carry that to the grave where it will be mocked, starved, dehydrated, beaten, suffocated and at left to die.

# Not Really Home Alone

While accountability is vital in our growth, it's only meant to augment the broader understanding with which God equips us about what He expects in our solitary Christian walks. Accountability is a way to huddle together to find warmth so when we're faced with decisions on our own regarding our individual battles against our entangling sins, we're fortified.

In a sense the things we learn through getting together with more mature believers who exhort, encourage and teach us become like an echo of grace when we're alone; God uses the wisdom they have shared to amplify His voice.

In between the times of being with those who advise us, God gives us help in ways that we wouldn't know how to ask from another human being. It's in those times, when we aren't walking closely with someone, that we learn to walk with God.

In those quiet times of obediently slogging along in repentance, meditating on His Word and His attributes, when no one is around, God can teach you lessons custom-made to deal with your unique issues. While there is no temptation that is not common to all humanity, you and I choose to sin for reasons that only we know (Prov. 14:10). Since God is the only one who truly knows our heart, then isn't it best to be in the silence with Him so He can perform surgery that will heal us. Our wounds, you know, are mortal, although thanks to God they aren't fatal.

In the end, God gives us the ability to build accountability with our brothers and sisters in Christ, but it's only so we can tear down the walls of sin we build against God. Accountability is a tool to help us grow out of our hatred of sin and increase in our love for God; though others may pour into us, God is the one who causes our growth (1 Cor. 1:13–17).

# The Things We Need As They Are Needful

I was 280 pounds, give or take, when I ran my first 5K. I'd signed up with some friends, fully intending to walk most of the way, but I found out from one of the team members: "No, we have to cross the finish line together *so you will run.*" There was no going back since I'd already committed, so with only five weeks to train for it, I did the only thing I could do and started running.

The thing was no one else on the team was training to run so I had to do it alone. Being as large as I was, it was hard to do, but what kept me going was the idea that I didn't have to do the race in record time, I just had to do it running. I learned all I could on my own by reading and asking people who were runners, and on the day of the race I told the rest of the team I would run, though it would be at my own pace, doing the best that I could.

The starting horn sounded and the large pack of runners slowly surged forward and I did too; head down as I determined to finish the race as I had trained. But as I looked to the side, one of my teammates, a handsome and athletic man who had formerly been on track in his younger days, trotted right beside me and said, "Would you like me to teach you how to breathe?"

From there he ran with me mostly step-for-step when he could have raced ahead. He taught me how to relax while I ran, he helped me slog through mud bogs, he kept me laughing when it was hard and when we came to the last crazy steep hill, he walked it with me. When the race ended, we did indeed all cross the finish line together as a team and I was pleased with myself for having run instead of walked. Yet I knew I hadn't done that race alone. I wouldn't have trained if I hadn't have been exhorted, and I might have given up in the face of the reality of the course if the more experience runner hadn't encouraged along the way. It's six years later and my running is forever changed because of them, especially because now I can actually do it where before I could only walk. While my encouragers don't go out with me when I run these days, they have taught me to always run my own pace with consistency and to do it breathing properly, reminding myself to relax.

God has signed us Christians up for this race and He expects us to run it to the best of our abilities. We may not be like my little friend who runs with a willing smile while her body screams to stop, at least not at first. But we have to start somewhere. We were designed to spiritually run and not be content to merely saunter. So let us go find those people who know how to run this race, so we can do our part more effectively.

We do this hard work with our hope anchored in our future home. In a little while, if we are faithful, when we have become stronger, we can become useful to others around us. Our transformation isn't for us alone, we've been saved for works specifically designed for us and it's only through being unhindered by sin that we can truly be ready to take on those jobs God has for us.

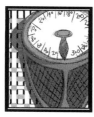

# Take A-Weigh

- We can't do this Christian walk alone for the long term.
- God provides people to help us battle our sin.
- Cherish the people in your life who say the hard things for your good.
- When you can't find accountability, seek to tighten your relationship with God.

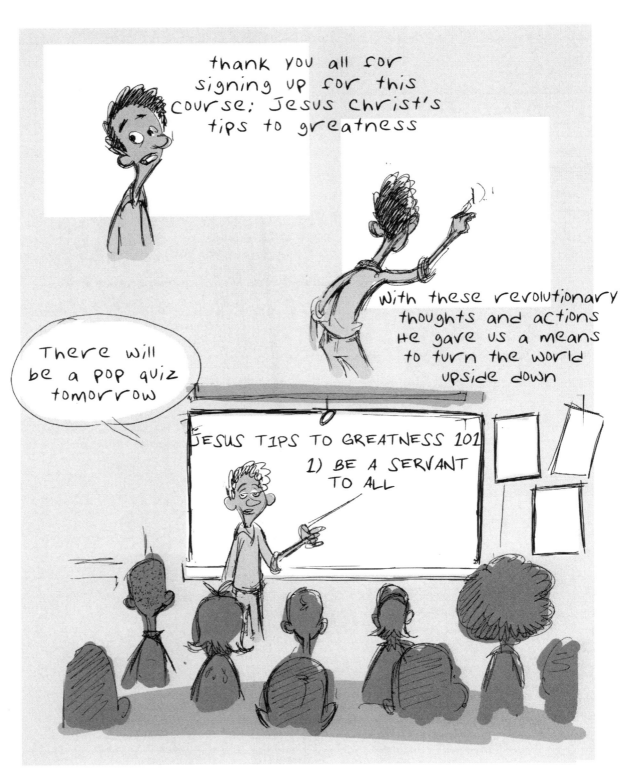

Mark 10:43-45

Chapter 15

# Set Free to Weed & Hoe

*Do nothing from selfishness or empty conceit, but with humility of mind regard one another as more important than yourselves; do not merely look out for your own personal interests, but also for the interests of others. Have this attitude in yourselves which was also in Christ Jesus, who, although He existed in the form of God, did not regard equality with God a thing to be grasped, but emptied Himself, taking the form of a bond-servant, and being made in the likeness of men.*     Phil. 2:3–6

She stood on the front porch of my house and announced she wanted to talk to me about the good news.

The woman was partnered with a young girl of eight or nine and I could tell by their clothing and the fact that there were other people walking in pairs along the street behind them that she and I had a different opinion of what the "good news" was.

That first time, I surprised her by being kind enough to let them inside, offer them both a cold glass of water, and eventually tell the little girl that they were in a cult. Over the next year and a half, while the woman surprised me by repeatedly returning, even though she knew that I was not going to yield, we did indeed talk about the gospel. Even though she was always with a different partner, once a month or so this sweet woman would return and we would talk, each of us trying to change the other's mind. There were times when I openly wept as I spoke of the true gospel, but she just took the elements of what I said, went home to research them and then returned the next time with reasons to refute them.

One day she came to the porch when I admit I wasn't as patient as I'd been on other occasions because I was cleaning my yard and was pressed for time. I didn't want to be dismissive, but I didn't want an hour and a half of conversation either, so I was perfunctorily polite as I continued to work on the same front porch where I'd met her nearly a year before. Somewhere in the course of our conversation, I mentioned my concept of repentant eating and she stopped as if someone had pressed her internal "pause" button.

"You mean the application of what you believe caused you to do this?" She said indicating the change she'd physically seen in me over the last year. She'd met me near the beginning of my highest weight and now she could see a powerful proof of the gospel that spoke more powerfully than my past words had done. She and her partner commented they never heard something like that before. I realized at that point, to that kind woman and her partner, their gospel was about doing good things in hopes of being one of the certain number of elect people to please their god, and here I was, someone who was quietly doing the hard work of turning her personal life over to God, knowing that I was already accepted by Him.

## Making It Not About You

At the beginning of the book, I talked about the gospel. I said it's the good news that there's a way to get to heaven. However the gospel isn't fully the gospel if that's all there is to it. The gospel must become the source of power in your life. It must change not only how you relate to God, but also your interactions with others. When you allow the gospel to have its full effect on your life, you become a powerful testimony of our invisible God.

Remember when I asked you why do you want to lose weight?

I've heard many specific reasons ranging from going to reunions, to getting back into high school clothes, to stopping the advancement of cancer. While these are fine reasons to do it, I hope that by now you understand the point of this book: that any reason to lose the weight for the sake of the weight loss alone is merely a smokescreen for the greater forest fire of repenting of the reasons why we exhibit long-term weight gain.

By now you understand you need to allow God to be the master of your life and to stop being a slave to food.

As I have said several times before, in this simple act of obedience we can be a living gospel tract that proves the reality of God. Yet if all we are is tacit displays of God's salvation, we're only fulfilling half our role as the redeemed church of Christ.

In the second phrase of His iconic prayer, Jesus taught His disciples to ask for God's Kingdom to come on earth as it is in heaven (Matt. 6:9–13). This request means both the asking for the literal coming of His actual Kingdom to replace this broken earth, as well as expecting to have our lives reflect everything that is entailed by being ruled even now by that eternal, mighty King.

If we're saved, then we all long for the day when God's actual Kingdom comes. So we live our lives in light of that hopeful expectation.

This means that when we start to lose this weight because of the hope of the gospel, our lives are not to be lived better now for ourselves alone. God has set us free from the chains of our sin for two reasons, to be like Him, and to serve Him by serving one another.

# In Service to the World

In the gospel according to Mark there was a man whom no one had been able to help because he was possessed by violent demons, but Jesus set him free. When the transformed man begged to come with Him on the rest of His travels, the Lord denied His request, telling him to instead stay at home and tell everyone of the hope found in really meeting God (Mark 5:18–20).

This world needs that kind of hope, even though right now they reject it.

Technology has given us things like light bulbs and telephones, but it's also given us the ability to see and learn everything there is to know in the world as well: the good, the bad, the perverted, the sorrowful and unjust, all pumped into our homes twenty-four hours a day in a relentless stream of darkness and despair.

Having access to everything at our fingertips from how to stuff a pheasant to seeing gruesome images of people killed by an extreme fundamentalist sect in some faraway land has made us smarter, but also weary and wary. Add to that humanity's love for their own personal sin, which causes them to shut out a good God so they can hold onto doing the evil they love, and you see this darkened world growing darker and darker.

Then along comes someone that believes there is a God who is going to bring an end to this evil world by replacing it with a holy one. Hope in this promise causes this person to surrender to this God's rule, and gradually their life shows the marks of knowing their new master. People in the dark world devoid of hope begin to take notice and they want to know what happened; they want to know why this person changed. Suddenly that person's obedient pattern of putting down the fork before overeating takes on a deeper meaning because he or she now has a platform that *proves* God is real!

Jesus said the entire message of God could be summed up in loving God with all that is in you and loving others as you love yourself (Matt. 22:36–40).

So in this we see that as we serve God by our obedience, we can also serve others by simply showing the effects of having obeyed. But what about the time before our pants begin to sag and people finally start to see cheekbones; what do we do in the meantime? While God is pleased that His children listen to His loving voice to repent of their sins He also expects them to live out "Thy Kingdom come" in their everyday lives by serving each other in His redeemed church.

# All That Extra Time

Before we repented of our greed and gluttony we may have spent a lot of time thinking about our food. If we weren't spending time planning our meals, then we were spending time eating.

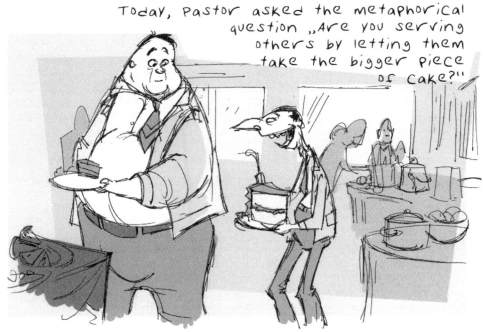

Today, Pastor asked the metaphorical question "Are you serving others by letting them take the bigger piece of cake?"

So I thought that during today's pot luck I'd give others a chance to practice that on me!

If we weren't spending time eating, then we were spending time thinking about *the next time we would eat*. We also spent a lot of money to make sure that we had the food that we loved to eat.

When we repent, we actually free up two things to use for God's service: time and money. Add to that the gift of energy. Now you and I have not only the resources to do what God commands, we also have the fortitude to do it as well.

The Bible commands us to serve one another, but so often we find that only a few of us obey God's edict. The reasons we give for our disobedience range from being too busy, to not feeling called, to being too introverted to reach out or too extroverted to take a lowly position. We don't know what our spiritual gifts are, or we don't possess enough education. Somehow we're always short on what we need, except excuses to not obey the command to serve. Whatever our reason for not doing what God commands with what He supplies, the truth is we're sinning if we don't serve in some way.

All of us are called to love, not just in word but also in truth and deed (1 John 3:17–18). The members of the early church could rely only on each other. Often when they became Christians they lost their property or were shunned by friends. Sometimes they were just very, very poor. Accordingly, members of the early church were instructed to do things like give of their resources or practice hospitality, not to show off their dishes and homes, but so that people could have their needs met. Some indeed were so helpless and alone they needed someone to care for them, while others needed someone to come along to comfort them in their intense persecution for their faith (Heb. 10:32–34; Rom. 12:13; James 1:27). Whatever the lack, the need was always found in turning for help to one another in the church body.

Sadly, in this present day in our Western culture, where we don't risk the loss of our property and for the most part the greatest attack to our reputations will be the snickers behind our backs, we can't find enough people to serve in the nursery changing poopy diapers and not enough people are willing to give up their daily coffee fix to set aside money to feed the hungry, let alone *actually roll up their sleeves to do it themselves*. There are fewer people interested in getting together to pray for the needs of the local body or the persecuted church than there are to discuss the newest series they binge-watched on pay-per-view. The single moms who lack life skills crack under the pressure while caring for little lives they need to shepherd all alone, and the widows and homebound sit in their houses as they listen to the monotonous tick tock, tick tock, tick tock of their clocks measuring the remains of their lives. The youths are no different, though they're too busy to hear the passage of time that they squander while in desperate need of someone to guide them in that phase of their lives when they may be shunning their parent's input. Then there's the sick, the marginalized and the people who need to learn but don't know where to turn, all of them missing out on the benefits of the service of others who have at least a little resource to fill someone else's needs.

We can all be selfish.

Just as the love of our pet sins like greed and gluttony blinds us to seeing the benefits of giving God our appetites, the lies that we believe that keep us from serving one another also keep us from learning the benefits of giving ourselves away to others as they have needs.

# The Lessons Learned by Loving Those Who Have Needs

God changes you in many ways while you learn to focus on others outside yourself. So what holds us back from serving? If it's not the reasons I mentioned earlier (which amount to justifications for our selfishness and laziness), it comes down to the fact that needy people are often a lot of work.

That's why they are needy . . .

However, God calls us to do it and gives us blessings in serving others. The first practical thing we gain when we give up our time is we have less time to willfully sin (Eph. 5:15–16). So many of us are sitting around bored, or hypnotized by the boob tube, or entangled by the World Wide Web while our hands mechanically go from the bag or bowl to our mouths and then back again. But now we, who understand that sport eating is sinful, can replace that sinful habit with the pursuit of God. We can trade in our self-service for serving others. Hooray! We can do this. It'll decrease the time we spend battling against our sin because while we're thinking of other's needs, we don't have time to dwell on the fact that we can't satisfy our carnal natures.

We also get the privilege of seeing God at work as He uses us. Not only are you obeying His command to serve others, you also may literally be an answer to someone's secret prayer. There are needs that are identified, like when someone sends around a clipboard to ask for sign-ups to watch the children for the parents' night out, but there are also unspoken needs so desperate that the one in need has no idea how to ask anyone for help, so all they can do is pray to God who knows how to fill their needs. When as servants we open our eyes to fill the needs that we can see, even when people aren't asking, we may unwittingly be the answer God intends to meet that person's deeper unspoken need.

Overall, serving others taps into a deep resource to find personal growth by meeting the needs of others, especially when we do it for people who can do nothing for us in return. In exchange for the investment of time, resources and maybe emotional input, we learn compassion, patience and tolerance. I'm not saying it isn't tiring or taxing, frustrating or inconvenient at times. I'm not saying it isn't often thankless or doesn't involve more investment than we had originally intended, but as we go to God to pray for those we're helping and get the extra resources we need, we get a glimpse of how much God loves us; we reflect on how their weakness mirrors our own weakness before God.

We learn to see past their needs to their humanity, and to view them the way we would desire to be seen in our own desperation. We must learn to look past the thought that their need may take a while to resolve or may be always there, and just serve them with the same attitude we apply to our own personal struggles, relying on God's grace for that day. God may have you in their life for a long time, or He may only have you there for only a short, intense period. Either way, be faithful to serve them with your resources, time or money and energy that you now have because He has freed you from your sin.

Avoid the traps of becoming cranky and crabby—or self-righteous, with the attitude of "look how amazing I am for helping you." Dodge the tyranny of looking at your wristwatch as if you had someplace else better to be. You'll lose the check-box attitude if you actually serve the person in front of you, not only looking at their humanity or reflecting on your weakness before God, but *showing those you serve your humanity as well.*

In this way you put your arm around them with a sense that you're both in it together instead of standing over them like some beneficent lord.

# Single-Face Servants

*Let love be without hypocrisy. Abhor what is evil; cling to what is good. Be devoted to one another in brotherly love; give preference to one another in honor; not lagging behind in diligence, fervent in spirit, serving the Lord; rejoicing in hope, persevering in tribulation, devoted to prayer, contributing to the needs of the saints, practicing hospitality.  Rom. 12:9–13*

While during the last supper Jesus called His disciples to love one another with an overflowing love, the Bible also acknowledges that sometimes that's going to be a bit of a challenge, and calls us to tolerate each other in brotherly affection (Eph. 4:3).

We come to serve people unconditionally, however sometimes the most loving thing we can do is help them understand the impact of their choices. While all our sins are forgiven in Christ, there are times that the consequences of hurt and broken relationships need to be addressed. Sometimes while we're serving someone we may need to do the hard task of confronting a brother or sister who has been irresponsible. However, remember the lessons of accountability—are they unruly, fainthearted or weak?—and apply your actions to those attitudes while you're serving them accordingly. In any event, your service shouldn't be predicated on their compliance to "cleaning up their sin"—unless the person is truly being an unrepentant knucklehead. Even that I say with humility as I remember how Robin fed, advised and encouraged me for many years before the light bulb of repentance in some areas finally winked on in my heart.

We're called to love each other truthfully. The main purpose in loving each other in truth isn't so we can blast one another into submission, but in the end to actually restore and sometimes build a relationship, so that the restored person can serve God and serve others in the church as well.

The Bible seems to acknowledge that people are not going to "get" one another all the time, but it doesn't give us an "out" when it comes to serving the difficult people in our lives. Instead it encourages us to tolerate one another in brotherly love, remembering that God called us and we are to be diligently preserving the unity of the Spirit (Eph. 4:1–3). With the reminder that He loved us first, God calls us to serve others.

In that final Passover Jesus served His disciples by washing their feet as an example of how they were to serve one another and teach others to serve. He washed their feet even though He knew that in just a few hours one would betray His friendship while another would betray His life. If the God of the universe who created feet could lower Himself to wash them, this gives us encouragement to debase ourselves to serve others.

The command to tolerate one another in brotherly love isn't Scripture's way of rapping you on the nose and saying "gut it out," nor is it a resigned sigh to grin and bear it because this all will eventually end (like when you can get off at your stop after sitting on an extremely crowded metro next to slightly odd person). No, since this metro ride is a lifelong one that only stops at the gates of heaven, God is asking for more than gritting our teeth or grinning when it comes to tolerance, He's asking us to remember His grace.

In the command to walk worthy of the manner in which we were called while showing tolerance for one another, being diligent to preserve the unity of the Spirit (Eph. 4:1–3), we're told to look at this person with their peccadilloes and preferences, qualities and quips, worries and wishes, and remember one thing: God has promised He will save both you and that person and He is committed to change you into the people He wants you to be. So He will stick with you both, despite the way you are acting, because God sees the magnificent work of art He will one day make of you.

Even while serving one another, like everything that we do in this life, we must keep in mind the message and hope of the gospel.

God's command to love one another is just that, to love one another, *not "some another."* We're in the church together, and sometimes we're all at different places. Some of us may be more advanced in Bible reading; some of us may be better at praying; some of us may be better at being hospitable. Rather than leaving those behind who aren't as strong at things that we're strong at doing, we need to link arms with them and encourage them.

So often our problems with other brothers and sisters in Christ result from the idea that they aren't where we think they should be. We believe they should be more gracious, they should be more kind, they should be more self-controlled, etc. You're right: what they should be is perfect and yet—so should you, but still God loves us all in the meantime. It will help us to serve all those in the church with tolerance when we remember that as once we were, so are those who get on our nerves, if they too are regenerated in Christ. If we meditate on just how much God loved us, loves us, and will always love us, we can find the "tolerance" to redirect that love to others in the family of Christ.

Now, I'm not saying we have to run out there and serve *only* the difficult people, or else we're Christian weaklings. Even Jesus seemed to click better with Peter, James and John so He took them on some special outings. What I am saying is if we serve only the people who come up to our standards of measurement, our growth will be less substantial than the growth we'll experience by forbearing challenging personalities.

When we prayerfully open ourselves to serving those people as they have needs, we'll become more patient and loving, more gentle and generous. Above all, we'll learn to see ourselves a little more clearly the way Christ sees us. Our friends love us because of our commonalities, but when we love others in the body of Christ who are challenging for us to love, we grow to have more in common with Jesus Christ who loved each person in His

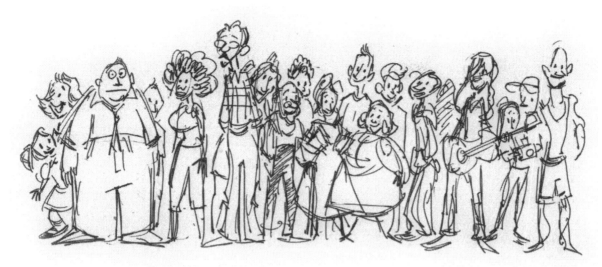

church enough to die for them when every one of us was still His enemy (Rom. 5:6–11).

So bearing this in mind we find the encouragement to serve ALL of God's "one anothers."

God equips us to serve individually but He also calls us to serve corporately as well. In either case we are to do it unconditionally and without a begrudging heart; we do it with love, and this is not just the warm squishy kind—we are to love the way God did when He sent His Son to die for us. (1 John 4:10-11)

# Even the Dung Beetle Has its Purpose

After reading this far in the book, by now you also understand how excited I am about the concept of having a relationship with God who personally deals with us as individuals, which is so much better than the mistaken idea that Christians should be stamped-out cookie cutter versions of each other with no trace of originality or imagination. It's not like God who created approximately 400,000 species of beetles was suddenly going to get tired when it came to redeeming the people of the earth. No, God gave us our personalities, our parents, our particular circumstances and the talents that have made us as different from one another as the cliché snowflakes.

And yet, we aren't clichés.

God wants to use our particular brand of theatrics to achieve His purpose in the world around us, so we needn't be ashamed for the things we have to offer. Not all of us are pastors, as Paul said in Ephesians—but not all pastors are artists either.

How do you discover what it is you're suited to do, so that you can serve?

To find where to serve corporately you need to ask yourself some questions. What do I like to do? What are my talents? What are my skills? What would I like to see changed? What injustices would I like to fight? At what do I excel? What are my useful assets?

The Westminster shorter catechism asks the question, "What is the chief end of man?"

The answer: "Man's chief end is to glorify God, and to fully enjoy him forever." If this is true, then the answers to those personal questions will apply those attributes and assets that make us unique to the sole purpose of glorifying God.

These were a few of the things I wrote down on my own list:

- I like to cook.
- I like to sew.
- I sing.
- I have no problem talking to strangers.
- I connect to high school students.
- I draw and do media things.
- I had a roommate who could get me plane flights for cheap.

I took account of these things as well as issues involved in my family of origin (i.e., from single-parent family, not married, with a newly gained understanding of my long-term weight issues as sin) and I asked myself how could I use these things in the church.

When I did this I learned that sometimes we don't have to attach ourselves to a ministry to serve with our gifts, we just have to open to serve wherever there's a need and do it!

Singing in the choir was a no-brainer since I was already doing it (more on that later) yet I felt because I'm single I could do more (1 Cor. 7:32). We have several ministries at the church I attend where I figured I could serve based on my assets and family history.

After being in the kitchen ministry for several events I decided it wasn't my thing. I'm not good in my own kitchen with other people around let alone being in a group kitchen where everyone is bumping into each other with dull knives while wanting to chat about deep personal issues.

So I tried the high school group. Since my church high school group was small, I found I really wasn't necessary. I wasn't needed as a small group leader. I wasn't needed for camp. What I ended up doing was teaching two girls how to sew. We spent six to eight weeks making dresses that probably were too complicated to teach two young women: but on the Saturdays when we struggled with the vintage patterns with instructions that read like someone wrote them who had never sewn before, we went from speaking about trivial things like geeky movies to the deep things of Christ. Not only that, after our sessions, when I brought the girls home, I learned some things from their mothers as well.

I wasn't a high school leader at first; I was just somebody who was teaching them how to sew. That would prepare me for several years later when I became an actual high school staff person at our church, when I combined my love of cooking, the fact I'm single and had the money, and that my heart broke for the need I saw in the girls to have unity among themselves. For a year I would have monthly lunches in my house where I would invite all the high school girls and any of their non-churched girlfriends to my home where I would cook them an elaborate meal and give them a place where they could actually encourage one another through conversation and games. At the end of our three hours, I'd share a devotional from the Bible on some aspect of unity and we'd break up into groups and pray for one another's needs.

Having a roommate who worked for the airlines was a fun perk and as she had grown up a missionary kid in the Philippines; she and I went back there to help her parents move and generally had a good time. I also went to Germany with plans to help some missionary friends and got to know some of the young Germans there.

The reason for sharing those experiences is to emphasize the point that we're made with specific jobs in mind. Just as the common brown dung beetle has one purpose and the colorful rainbow stag beetle has another, we may be male or female, black, white, brown, red or yellow—but our uniqueness defines us more than our common humanity. The very thing that annoyed me in one ministry, the interaction with the people, was the very thing that I loved about another, the interaction with people who were high school kids and people in other countries. I wouldn't have learned that if I hadn't tried on the ministries like a person would try on clothes in a dressing room.

In the end, finding a place to serve is a process, one you won't discover if you don't do it. Really, serving should be as easy as filling a need when its expressed, but what do we do when needs aren't expressed? Does that mean we just sit around doing nothing? ("WAHOO! IT'S ALL ME! Welcome to the ME show! Now hand me that bowl of popcorn!") If that's how you feel, then you get what you want: fat, bored or lonely. The ministry of ME leaves you empty. We were made for God's purposes and we need to find and fulfill them.

# Sometimes the Only Equipment You Need is a Willing Heart

Bear this in mind: just because you're gifted in something, doesn't mean it's always needed. Serve anyway! I recently went on a short term mission trip where they needed a man to teach some pastors to be better pastors, some women trained in counseling to teach the women about relationships, construction people to help build a library, a person to teach the choir, and an assistant to help him, a person to teach guitar, and a high school person to document the work the team was doing. What they didn't need was an artist. The only job they had left was for someone to put sticky book covers on the books in a library to protect them.

I struggled with that. I thought I was so much better than covering books. But the God of the universe, who had spoken the trees into existence, came to earth where He used tools to make tables; how beneath Him was that job? A friend reminded me of the widow who gave her two mites and no one else saw her sacrifice but Jesus alone (Mark 12:41–44),

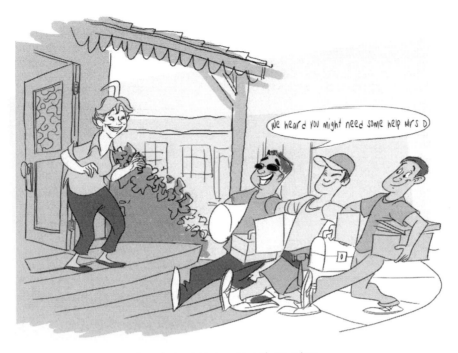

Service never goes out of style.

encouraging me that any service, no matter how small, that's rendered to God, is pleasing to Him. Don't overlook being the one who puts away the folding chairs or cleans off the tables or invites people over for dinner who may be just passing through town. Don't overlook meeting new people in your church and asking them to lunch. These may not be "ministries" but you are ministering; you're showing love to one another, showing preference to one another, and serving one another.

It's said that in churches 20 percent of the people are doing 80 percent of the work. I'd like to hope it's not because we're lazy, but just because we don't know what to do. Now you know—go do something! If that doesn't work, go do something else. But don't do "nothing."

You don't have to be perfect, just willing.

## The Unintended Spotlight

I'd been a Christian for a long time before I finally submitted my appetite to God. During that time I had served in the choir at my church. I believe that though that's not leadership in the strictest sense of the word, still being up there in front of people shows the congregation "Follow me as I follow Christ." Well, leading up to my change of heart, I realized I was doing wrong but I didn't want to change, so I stepped away from choir for a number of years. Three months after I started my repentant eating, a new friend suggested out of the blue:

"You should join the choir."

"I have stuff," I demurred referring to my growing awareness of my greed as sin. "But thank you, and please pray for me."

He stared at me flatly and replied, "Carole, you should join the choir."

I thought maybe I wasn't clear so I iterated my former statement with slightly different words . . . or maybe not; I can't remember; it might have just been *more* words. This time my friend said, with matter-of-fact indifference, "Are you working on your stuff? We all have stuff. You should join the choir."

I realized I actually was working on my stuff, and though God called me to be perfect, perfection takes time (2 Cor. 3:18). So I joined the choir.

Serving while repenting gives you the opportunity to proclaim God's goodness and rule in your life in ways you would never have had by staying on the sidelines. Though God commands us to be perfect as He is perfect, He knows we're weak flesh that's why He tells us to confess our sins and He will cleanse us. You may be as I was, and think you've got to be perfect now or else you can't serve Him. Remember though, God doesn't see as man sees, God sees your heart.

If your heart is submitted to His will, then He'll bring the perfecting, as you keep submitting. I didn't know it at the time, but my life became an encouragement to others as I stood up there in the choir loft and the members of the congregation actually saw evidence of my weight loss as a consequence to my submission to Christ. They saw it and asked how I was doing it. Each time I got a fresh opportunity to talk about the things God taught me through His Word. Each time He's gotten the glory as I've continually submitted to His will.

For a bonus, here's a thought: serving others helps you lose weight. Conventional wisdom tells you to do things like take the stairs instead of the elevator or park at the outside of the parking lot at the store, but let me put this in your mind hamper. Try losing the words, "Would you do me a favor and—" if it means doing it for yourself, which will make you move more. That's one of the things I made a decision to do early on.

Quit asking people to serve you, in fact, be the one who hops up first when someone asks for help or needs someone to run an errand. Not only will you bless them, you'll burn more calories. And here's the more important thing—you'll get to practice treating others as more important than yourself. As you do this in the little things it'll become second nature for you to be the first one to hop up and take someone's plate to the kitchen or bend over and pick up the newspaper from the driveway for your friend you're coming to visit instead of stepping over it. In due time God will give you greater opportunities to serve others—*and burn calories at it!* So everybody wins!

# Community Gardens

In the end, serving one another builds unity and while it's God's command to prefer others above ourselves, the benefit we get from serving sacrificially is we become a part of the community of Christ and as part of that community, people learn to watch out for you.

Without people to watch out for us we can continue to sin in our solitude, which further separates us from one another and builds walls against God. We make a choice when we don't serve others—we serve ourselves as we fortify the personal kingdoms we should be striving to destroy.

In my neighborhood are two community gardens: beautiful lots that contain both vegetables as well as some flowers. I've never been a part of a community garden, but I have long admired them. I'm not committed enough to turn my back yard into a farm (I like my grass too much), so the idea of having someplace else to go and grow vegetables appeals to me, not quite enough for me to join one, but enough for me to admire the gardens as I pass them on my morning runs.

In thinking about service as part of a community in the context of the church, I could see there were benefits similar to those of working in a community garden. Beyond receiving fruit from your labor, here are some additional perks of serving in your church:

- Serving in the local church brings various people together from different backgrounds (differing ages, races, cultures, social classes).

- Serving in the local church helps us grow in understanding our identity as Christians.

- Serving in the local church increases our sense of community as a church.

- When people serve in the local church, they stay "in the loop" of community activities and issues.

- Serving in the local church trains leaders to lead and people to be humble.

- Serving in the local church provides a defense against false teachers coming in and deceiving people. When people are a community, no one is lonely and vulnerable.

- Having more people serving in the local church means more people are in the building more of the time, in case some threat arises.

- A church community that serves together is warm and welcoming to newcomers instead of intimidating. This can be like a magnet for nonbelievers, including those from other cultures.

- Serving in the local church meets the specific needs in the church body, as well as the needs of sister churches and the local community outside the church walls.

- Serving in the local church provides people who don't have goods, food or company to be helped by people who have those things to give.

- Serving in the local church allows people to work side by side with the common goal of building the body of Christ without speaking the same language.

- Serving in the local church gives retirees the opportunity to be useful when they still have the energy and health to work.

- Serving in the local church helps bridge the gap between younger and older people.

- Serving in the local church is a healthy, free activity for youth that helps them grow in a physically productive way with eternal benefits.

- Serving in the local church gives meaning to lives that would otherwise be dismissed as useless.

- Serving in the local church provides a retreat from the world into the encouraging company of like-minded believers.

- Serving in the local church provides a means to flesh out the biblical command to not only hearers of the word but also doers of it (James 1:22).

When God set you free from the chains of your sin, He unlocked the treasure chest of the endless possibilities of what time, money and energy can accomplish. Part of the process of growth involves not only sharing with others the deep places of your heart, but also your transformed life. It may not involve having deep conversations; it might just be as simple as bringing someone a meal when they're sick or helping an overwhelmed clutter-oh-holic clean their house. There are always many needs to be filled around you.

We in the modern the church can tend to drift, whether it's from relationship to relationship or congregation to congregation. We're restless and discontented. We sit in the pews in our invisible bubbles of space, filled with resentment, judgments, selfishness, and sheer laziness, daring others to come near. We need to understand that we are the solution to the problem we see. We need to serve each other from the heart for the cause of Christ. We need to pop those bubbles and move closer to one another. Don't be discouraged if your advances aren't immediately reciprocated. Have patience and pray for those who are slow to thaw. Be diligent. Start tearing down the kingdom of yourself, and in time, you'll have so little lonely time (as it's filled with others) that you won't have as much time to be stuffing your face with food because you're lonely or sad.

Now . . . about all that tasty food you have to control yourself around after getting invited to all those dinners of the new people in your life, well, that's your own look-out.

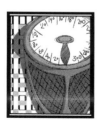

# Take A-Weigh

- God set us free from our sin and given us resources to serve one another.

- We can overcome challenges to serving one another by remembering that God saved us when we were "challenging."

- Figure out what you enjoy doing and find places to serve doing it.

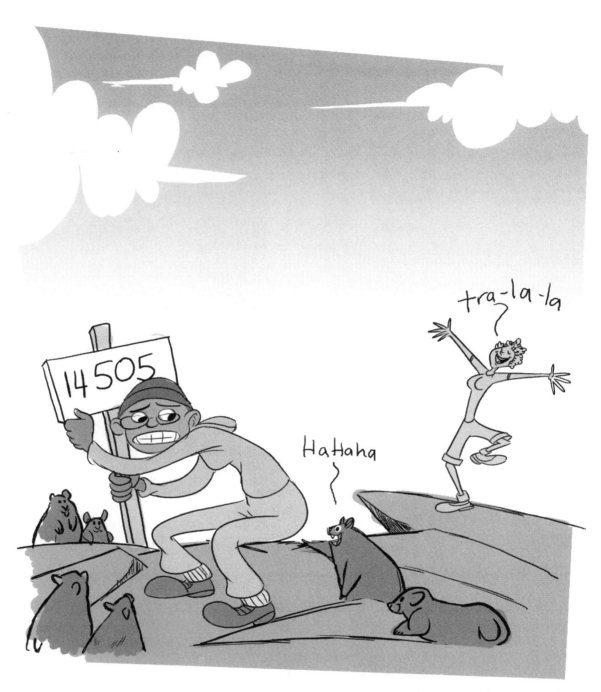

I had not expected the tallest peak in the contiguous united states to be so high... or have so. Many. Marmots.

# Near & Far Peaks
## My UN-Epilogue

William Shakespeare asked the question through the lips of a love struck teenage girl, "What's in a name?" Names, titles, and brands have the power of story. A good one can inspire action, thought, or change. A mediocre one can only rouse the passions of your friends and family out of mild interest and support.

I tried a boatload of titles before I settled on "The Food Ain't the Problem." Each one was close, but none of them captured both the content of the book as well as its tone. After three weeks of trying I drew my line in the sand and chose a title.

My friends had other ideas.

They pushed, prayed and put their head's together with me to come up with something better than what I thought was "perfect."

Their insistence was frustrating. I figured I had something. My new title was better than what I had before which was "God's Itty Bitty Fat Book." That title which, while catchy, neither compellingly represented the content of the book nor was true because at over two hundred and seventy pages there was nothing remotely "itty bitty" about it.

Eventually my friends' loving insistence broke through my "perfect" title and led me to the one I have now. Like dominoes, the remaining pieces that I struggled to create fell into place as the external look of my book was wrapped up in a pretty red bow.

God, in His kindness, gives me pictures through my pain or frustration—illustrations to teach me the way my mind works. This final story of a "title found" gave light to the idea that we can be blind to the right way because we think we've found *the* perfect way.

We can do this when tackle our destructive habits like the one mentioned in the pages of this book. We settle for our idea of the perfect and miss out on the truth.

# A View of the Summit From the Road to It

In the process of finishing this book, I finally had my visit to Mount Whitney. While I was there, my hiking partner asked me what was next for me now that my journey of training for this event was being consummated. Was it a marathon or some other great physical challenge? I told her it was time for me to finish revising this book, for that was as difficult as the many miles I'd run, heavier than all weights I'd lifted, and more grueling than any of the mountains I'd climbed. It was particularly challenging to wrap up the writing because I didn't know what my last words should be—and frankly, because I'm not good at following through with things to the end. Most of all, I felt I wasn't qualified to speak on the subject because I was having difficulty getting off the last few pounds.

So a few days after doing the greatest thing I'd ever done as a woman afraid of heights and formerly fat, I thought of God's character in light of the great mountain I'd just summited. Indulge me these last stories and in the end I will glean for you some hope as you set out on your journey of obedience.

You'd think that with it being the tallest mountain in the contiguous United States, you'd be able to see it from the freeway. Although it stands 14,505 feet above sea level, it's not easily spotted amidst the Sierra's peaks. In fact, from the city of Lone Pine, the first mountain you see is not Mount Whitney but Lone Pine Peak, which is why the people who discovered Lone Pine Peak mistakenly thought that IT was the tallest mountain in California. Driving up to it, Whitney doesn't look that big either. I told my friend I thought it looked doable, and she smiled and commented that my perspective on what was doable had changed from all my training. I don't know if my perspective had changed or if I just couldn't comprehend how big Whitney really was because I had no scope. I wonder if I would have thought the same if I had been able to see the mountain more prominently from the freeway and all alone?

Such is with God. He's far more enormous than we think He is, and there are so many other things that compete with Him that we perceive to be bigger than He is because of our perspective. This is the trap of only focusing on what's right in front of us instead of what we must take in faith as truth.

Whitney is the tallest mountain in the contiguous United States not because I can see it in comparison to others—Whitney is the tallest *because it is*.

Likewise, God is bigger than anything else we desire in our lives. We think that other things are bigger than He is: other people, other loves, and other passions. We pursue those other "peaks" in our lives because we can't see God for who He truly is from our vantage point. Therefore it becomes a trial and error summiting adventure as we climb one peak after another trying to find meaning and purpose in our lives. Each time we accomplish that task we realize it wasn't the answer and we're left discouraged and tired if we don't remember the hope found only in the love of God.

The Bible speaks of a day when the mountains will be laid low (Isa. 40:4) and likewise all the things in this life will be laid low and we will see God for who He really is. For now, we must battle with our false perspective of Him. We must not give up when we discover we've wandered off onto another peak. When we see we've been misdirected, we must return to learning about God with the same energy we pursued whatever misguided peak we traversed, but be encouraged by this: Comprehending an infinite God will take a lifetime. We'll never be able to take Him in, in all His grandeur, in one sitting. We must approach God the way you approach a massive mountain: with faithfulness, dedication, and a long-term commitment.

To get to understand God, who is the peak above all peaks, you must commit to walk with Him. When you do, you learn Him step by step. He's not at all who we think He is. Whitney wasn't at all what I thought it was. I thought it was the pictures I'd seen of it in the books and Internet blogs: the hard impassive peaks that shoot up like granite teeth that hold no life because they can support no trees. Why do people focus only on the granite? Because of what I'd seen, I was fearfully prepared for the effort, but only for the effort. I didn't know what truly lie in store for me.

The Whitney I experienced didn't look like those pictures. As I followed the marked trail, I saw life, I saw beauty, and I saw wonder. Sure it was a long ascent, but there was so much to captivate my attention that it took my mind off the painful effort. Like Whitney, there's a trail to get through God's heart. It's not so difficult that it can't be done, but you have to want to do it, and as you put in the work to walk through the Mountain that is God Himself, you see so many beautiful things. He is not all granite and angst. If you seek Him respectfully, like the mountain you'll be safe to traverse Him. You'll be safe and you'll find joys that exceed your puny paltry self-assumed understanding of Him. God is alive.

Mount Whitney was alive with the sounds of water everywhere, places you could see and places you could only hear. It was living and transforming as the elements affected it. We saw a rockslide happen right before our eyes and the mountain was not the same for us as it was for the people who'd passed it just five minutes before us. There was hidden beauty of mirrored lakes that reflected the mountain's trees and skies above them, and the various climates created by its individual areas fostered different environments for flora to grow that wouldn't have grown around the bend before it. The mountain kept changing with every step. Well, not so much every step, but every mile. There was a different thing to see.

That's the same with God. We have to keep walking with Him, keep walking through Him. If we do, we'll find so much more beauty than we ever could imagine.

The book I bought on Whitney could only tell a tiny bit of what it was to hike it. It could only tell you with its printed words how to prepare how to ascend it. It was one author's experience in climbing it, and in the end, it wasn't anything to compare to actually doing it for myself. The Bible is the same way. Although God told the writers what to write about Him, even still it's just a poor copy of who God really is. But it's all we have. It's the road map through His heart, and one day we'll see the summit of Him. So since it's all we have, we need to acquaint ourselves with what we can about Him through its pages. As we carefully pick our steps across His streams, we need to let our eyes of awe behold the majesty of God's hidden beauty. We must not ever become complacent to think because we've understood one part of Him in the meadow, that we understand Him in the ravines. No, God is alive. Therefore our perspectives of Him will change, and this living, large and loving God will transform *us* as we apprehend Him step-by-step, mile-by-mile.

The state of Colorado boasts multiple peaks that tower over 14,000 feet but they still fall short of California's Mount Whitney as the tallest in the nation. There can only be one tallest.

So you see, that's why I say this isn't a diet book. It's a book about how God is real, so real that even the food I eat is submitted to Him. The consistency of how faithful I am to God defines my success or failure over time, but it doesn't define how much He loves me—He gave up His Son to me show that.

In the end, though you may lose a few or many pounds as you apply the principles from this book—the weight along the way is more like the vistas I saw on all the mountains: They weren't the end. Even reaching the top of Whitney wasn't the end. The end was when I'd gotten home, exhausted, beaten up, but happy for the experience of having seen the whole job through to its completion.

In this life where God's goal is to conform us to the image of His Son, there will always be work. Just as I stumbled and fell on the many mountains I hiked in my training time, I always got up and kept going because the "done" of having finished Whitney was the goal.

What is your done? Is it your weight number? Is it a relationship you hope to gain, or a position you hope to attain? Be careful you're not climbing Lone Pine Peak instead of God who really matters.

In this book, I've often addressed both the nonbeliever and the Christian, but the sad thing for me is that if you've made it this far in the book and you're still a nonbeliever, your eyes aren't capable of seeing the real tallest mountain peak at all.

If you made it to the end of the book and you're still a nonbeliever, then that's all you have—your lesser peak of weight loss. And while it's a notable goal, it's an empty one at best. Any number of events in your life can derail you and sap you of your motivation to go on . . . and make you end up back at the foot of the mountain of your struggle with weight, only worse: farther down, having fallen there with a shameful kerplunk.

If you're a Christian: the weight is only *a consequence* of having your "done" mean the completion of standing blameless before God your Father. Not blameless because you were perfect at eating the right portion sizes, but blameless because God rendered you so through Jesus.

That's the hope when I fail. That's the call that drives me to get up and slay my grumbly will (which at this moment wants a burrito from the taco shack down the street, though I've already eaten dinner). It isn't so I can lose the weight—but because I want to look like Jesus when I stand before the Father. I want to stand there not merely as "a perfect size six," but as someone who's glorified in a way that only will be known when all God's children stand before Him unashamed.

God who is the light of heaven stands at the ready for all who come to Him, and that's the hope and joy that should drive us past the thought, "ugh, I blew it again."

As the current popular saying goes "The struggle is real . . ."

. . . The weakness we will always have with us—but we who have Jesus will also have Him there as well. A Christian lives not for the "done" of this life but the "well done" when we stand at last before the Father.

## At the Crossroads

The beginning of this journey is to submit to God as your master. If that's not your main focus, then anything you do after that just replaces the god of results for the god of your appetite. In the end, we need to give up everything, even our expectations of a peaceful, healthy and happy life: "...in view of the surpassing value of knowing Christ Jesus my Lord, for whom I have suffered the loss of all things, and count them but rubbish so that I may gain Christ" (Phil. 3:8.) As I've said throughout the pages of this book, all of those other things are merely temporary.

We need to value Him above everything we desire most.

Just before He was to be crucified, a woman came to Jesus while He was attending a dinner party, bringing with her a jar of perfume worth a year's salary. She broke the jar and poured it on His feet, wiping them with her hair as a show of extravagant worship. As the aroma of this valuable offering filled the room, some of his disciples complained that she'd wasted her money, saying that instead it should have been sold and they could have given the money to the poor. Jesus' response was not to rebuke the woman, but to remind the men what was important. *"Why do you bother the woman? For she has done a good deed to Me. For you always have the poor with you; but you do not always have Me"* (Matt. 9:10–11).

We will always have struggles in this life, as long as we are affected by the world and our sinful desires. The only hope we have, then, is that the Savior who loved us while we were yet His enemies will love us when we fail.

Someone recently asked me online how to keep the weight off once we're done losing it.

I told her I didn't completely have a handle on it since I wrestle back and forth with about twenty-five pounds. I told her it was important to keep striving anyway because that's what marks a believer: our perseverance and our hope in His forgiveness and His grace. Life isn't easy. We won't be perfected this side of heaven. I think God allows the struggles in our lives to keep us humbly clinging to Him.

That last statement doesn't make Him a sadist, but someone who understands what we really need is not to be done, but to be with Him. That's when we're done. Our "done" is really a shallow vision, like a child's drawing of pony is laughable compared to Ruben's majestic painting of a horse.

I said from the beginning that this isn't a diet book. If all you got from it was how to lose weight, then you've missed the point. Everything I've written about all that I've learned in the past six years from this weighty journey has been about how God is more real than everything, and my relationship with Jesus is what I truly need. So even when I fail and gain a little weight, or think an inappropriate thought or mistreat someone instead of being kind or just act like a plain old sinful human being, I don't give up in my struggle. I return to strivng to obey God.

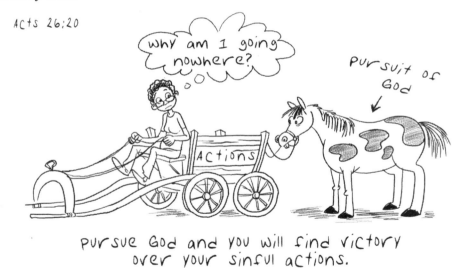

pursue God and you will find victory over your sinful actions.

## The Un-Ending

It's only fitting to call this an U*n*-Epilogue in my non-diet weight loss book. An epilogue means the concluding speech, the end. However, for a Christian whose life is a series of steps in sanctification, there really is no end this side of death until we finally hear the words, "Well done, good and faithful servant, you may enter your rest."

Only God can perform the final epilogue.

I guess in this my final words to you, that is what I would focus on: the idea that there's no rest in this battle against sin this side of the "well done." We'll find times where we're tremendously vigilant and other times we'll struggle to clamber out of the pit into which we fell when we were being wantonly rebellious. We have a great hope, though, for we find it in the loving grace of God our father. One day in heaven we will be finally free of the sins that so easily entangle us. They will have no hold on us because we'll be in the presence of God and He'll be so much more amazing than anything we could sinfully desire for ourselves.

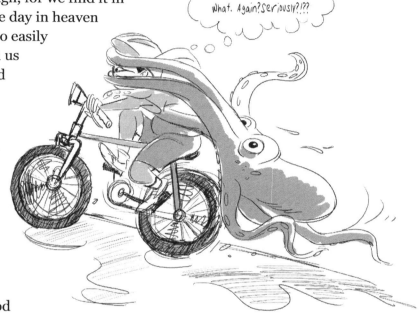

What it's like when exercise becomes a drag.

Let this be an encouraging reminder when you, like me, must repeat the cycle of repent, obey, deny yourself, fail, get up and start all over again. We tend to measure our achievements by having accomplished them but we don't at all value the concept of attempting them. We need to remember that the sins God indicates we should rout from our lives wouldn't even be in our radar to attack had not He let us know they were wrong in the first place. Therefore it's the living to please Him no matter how hard the battle, no matter how many times you fail, that's the accomplishment. It proves you're alive to keep fighting! Those who are dead won't live to please the Lord. They can't even try (Rom. 8:5–8).

So we who belong to the Lord need to look beyond the peaks of the weight lost or the marriage saved or the stolen goods returned or whatever other victories over sin we have accomplished. Those are *great* things, but when we struggle and fail and the goal seems so far away we get discouraged and want to give up; we forget we're on the mountain and the journey will not be complete until we're home. It may be a rough hike, but we need to keep going.

In the end—or at least along the way to the end, we may reach our goal of that exact magical number on the scale, but it won't count in God's record book. He isn't looking for people who've accomplished much by their perfected their bodies; He's looking for people who have lived their lives with the hope to finally be with their heavenly Father.

If you are a nonbeliever, I can only plead with you to come to Jesus for your salvation.

We'll all stand before the judgment seat of God one day and your accomplishments, no matter how grand they are, will be completely inadequate in comparison to the perfection that is only found in Jesus Christ.

But—

To the believer who views God's call to perfection as daunting, take heart. I write these final words of encouragement to you. When we come before God after a lifelong pursuit of what He defines as perfection, we will be warmly greeted like the child who shows his puny arm muscle and says, "Look how big I am!" Then God like an earthly father who sees his child's tiny muscle with eyes of love, will accept us. For it is by His grace we have been made strong. It is by His grace that we have been with Him from all along. On that day, after a lifetime of striving, we will finally be able to enter into our rest. For now, we keep on running, working, obeying, loving and pressing on to the upward call of God in Christ Jesus (Phil. 3:14). It's my hope that the words of this book have in some small way turned your eyes from your "perfect way" to the right way: God's hidden path to truth (Matt 7:13-14).

Well, I guess I better stop now and go for a walk or something. God bless you as you seek God and learn to be like Him. And may you trust Him for the results of weight loss in His perfect timing. I know I am.

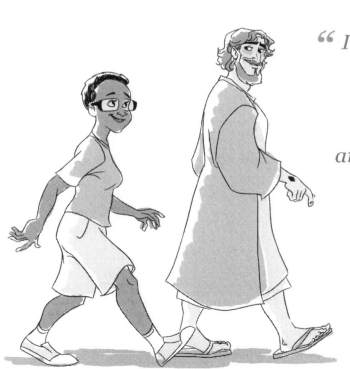

*Jesus said to them,*
*" I am the bread of life;*
*he who comes to Me*
*will not hunger,*
*and he who believes in Me*
*will never thirst. "*

*John 6:35*

Printed in Great Britain
by Amazon